Dental Practice

Get in the Game

DENTAL PRACTICE

GET IN THE GAME

Edited by

Michael Okuji, DDS, MPH, MBA
Group Director, General Clinic
Academic Administrator, Division of Restorative Dentistry
School of Dentistry
University of California, Los Angeles
Los Angeles, California

Quintessence Publishing Co, Inc
Chicago, Berlin, Tokyo, London, Paris, Milan, Barcelona,
Istanbul, Moscow, New Delhi, Prague, São Paulo, and Warsaw

Library of Congress Cataloging-in-Publication Data

Dental practice : get in the game / edited by Michael Okuji.
p. ; cm.
Includes bibliographical references and index.
ISBN 978-0-86715-492-4
1. Dentistry--Practice. I. Okuji, Michael.
[DNLM: 1. Practice Management, Dental--United States. WU 77 D4135 2009]
RK58.D447 2009
617.60068--dc22
2009050545

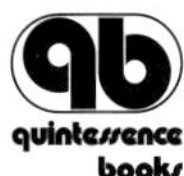

Quintessence Publishing Co Inc
4350 Chandler Drive
Hanover Park, IL 60133
www.quintpub.com

Editor: Lisa C. Bywaters
Cover and internal design: Gina Ruffolo
Production: Sue Robinson

Printed in Canada

Contents

Preface

The single most important step in a career in dentistry is to serve the public by establishing your first practice. It is an action that creates the possibility for professional growth and personal fulfillment. Thus, I focused on two major goals in writing this book: *(1)* Preparing senior dental students and recent graduates for entry into the practice of dentistry, and *(2)* providing relevant information in an easily accessible format.

For some time I pondered the idea of training students to become dental health practitioners in this era beset with ramifications unlike any experienced in former times. The now outdated model in which fees for services were paid directly to the dentist by the patient served practitioners well in the past and enabled them to maintain their offices as well as their families. However, this era of simplicity came to a close decades before the end of the 20th century. Events during this first decade of the 21st century have further convinced me that the business side of dental practice needs specific emphasis in the dental curriculum.

This book is meant for true beginners in the business of dentistry. It is not required that readers of this book possess previous business experience or have a family member already in the field of dentistry. Every effort has been made to emphasize the fundamental issues in the startup of a dental practice using easy-to-read, informative guidelines without ponderous fluff. I have included key points and terms in the margins to reinforce important concepts and for easy reference; in addition, online resources are presented (as indicated by the mouse icon in the margin) to allow the reader to access additional information. This is done, however, with the caveat that some links may no longer be valid at the time of reading.

The range of topics is not intended to be exhaustive or perfect, and I do not claim to have presented any "new" knowledge. However, by collaborating with colleagues who understand the rigors of making decisions in a climate of uncertainty and incomplete knowledge, I am able to offer the reader a compilation of experiences garnered over the years and condensed into a single source. Each contributor has personal experience in both private practice ownership and practice management education.

It is also important to point out that the book is not intended to substitute for legal, accounting, insurance, and commercial advice. Rather, it is meant to provide pertinent information that will equip students and graduates with basic tools to understand business concepts and vocabulary in order to ask appropriate questions. It is worth remembering that success and happiness are not guaranteed by the lawyer, accountant, or business advisor; they offer advice and recommendations–nothing more.

The future is yours to make. Good fortune to all.

Acknowledgments

I am indebted to the book's contributors, whose expertise illuminates pertinent aspects of the business side of dentistry. I am heartened by their willingness to give precious time to this project.

On a personal level, I am inspired to venture into the literary thicket by my mentor, Distinguished Emeritus Professor Clifton O. Dummett, DDS, MSD, MPH, of the University of Southern California. A now-retired teacher, orator, and administrator, Dr Dummett's prolific scholarly writings–scientific, historical, and commentary–represent a major contribution to the dental literature. I am grateful for my friendship with Clifton and Lois Dummett and for their encouragement.

My heartfelt appreciation to Tomoko Tsuchiya, Vice President of Quintessence Publishing Company, for her faith and confidence in my book proposal and her steady hand to guide a novice author. Gloria Vo-Truong and Rouzan Kheranian lent invaluable assistance to the tedious chore of fact checking. However, any error of fact, omission and commission, remains solely with me.

Contributors

Frank Licari, DDS, MPH, MBA
Professor and Associate Dean of Academic Affairs
College of Dental Medicine–Illinois
Midwestern University
Downers Grove, Illinois

Richard Nathan, DMD, MS
Associate Clinical Professor
Department of Orofacial Sciences
Division of Periodontics
School of Dentistry
University of California, San Francisco
San Francisco, California

David Okuji, DDS, MBA
Clinical Instructor, Pediatric Dentistry
General Practice Dental Residency
Cambridge Health Alliance
Boston, Massachusetts

Michael Okuji, DDS, MPH, MBA
Group Director, General Clinic
Academic Administrator, Division of Restorative Dentistry
School of Dentistry
University of California, Los Angeles
Los Angeles, California

Francis Serio, DMD, MS, MBA
Associate Dean for Clinical Affairs
School of Dentistry
East Carolina University
Greenville, North Carolina

Scott Stafford, DDS, MBA
Clinical Assistant Professor and Program Director
Practice Dynamics Division
Department of General Dentistry
Dental School
The University of Texas Health Science Center at San Antonio
San Antonio, Texas

Eric Studley, DDS
Clinical Associate Professor
Cariology and Comprehensive Care
College of Dentistry
New York University
New York, New York

Choosing a Path

David Okuji, DDS, MBA

As a dental student or recent graduate, you're about to enter the game of your lifetime . . . the practice of dentistry. As in any game, you will have to plan your strategy. Your challenge is to create and implement a career strategy that optimizes your goals and objectives and fits your personal skill set and the external environment in which you operate. Are you entrepreneurial? Are you managerial? Are you a "people person"? Is it important to live near your family and old friends? Do you want to live in Chicago or Smallville, Beverly Hills or Green Acres? Is earning a lot of money critical to your vision? Is having a lot of free time to pursue other activities important to your lifestyle? How many dentists are in the same location where you want to practice? The answers to these questions and myriad others like them help to assess personal skill and desire along with the external constraints and hurdles to becoming a player in the game. This chapter will help you give such questions thoughtful consideration, allowing you to formulate a strategy that will fit your personal vision and lead you down a successful career path.

Also included in this chapter are brief vignettes in which the contributing authors of the book describe their first job and the ways in which it influenced their eventual career path. These stories, along with the rest of the material in this chapter, are meant to encourage you to open your mind to the many opportunities available to you and to prepare you for finding your first job. Even as the main text encourages you to create a careful game plan, the stories will keep you grounded in the reality that winning the game requires the skill and agility to adapt to the state of play at any given time.

Goals and Objectives
Financial
Geographic
Temporal
Internal Resources
Clinical competency
Managerial skills
Entrepreneurial skills
Financial resources
CAREER
STRATEGY
External Environment
Competition
Consumer market
Financial market
Labor market
Government regulation

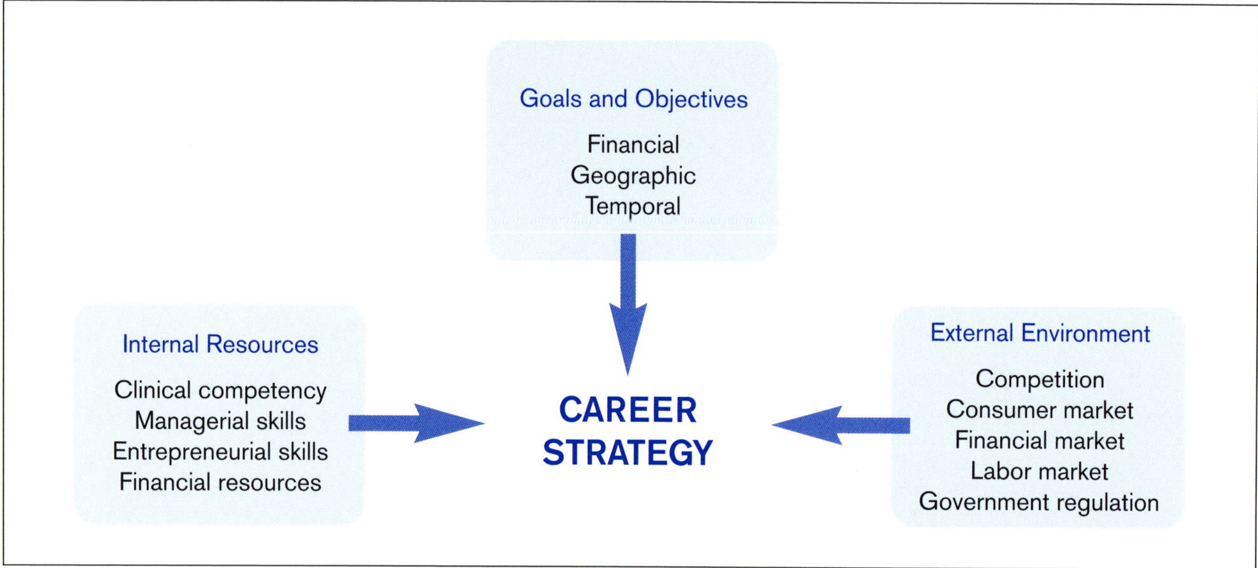

Fig 1-1 Three-pronged approach to a career strategy.

Career Strategy

There are three pieces that fit together to create your career strategy: your goals and objectives, internal resources, and the external environment (Fig 1-1).

Goals and Objectives

There are three types of goals and objectives: financial, geographic, and temporal.

Financial goals and objectives

Accumulating wealth over time in order to reach financial independence is the most common financial goal and objective. Therefore, what you must determine is how much wealth you need to accumulate to achieve the degree of financial independence you desire at the age at which you desire it.

Accumulation of wealth

net worth
Your assets minus your liabilities at any given point in time.

Your wealth, or net worth, is defined as your assets (ie, what you own) minus your liabilities (ie, what you owe) at any given point in time. If, on January 1, 2050, a dentist owns a home worth $2 million with an investment portfolio valued at $4 million and owes $1 million for a real estate loan, the wealth (net worth) equals $5 million as of January 1, 2050.

You accumulate wealth through income from: *(1)* direct effort (eg, being paid a wage of $500 per day as an associate dentist); *(2)* the work of others (eg, employing an associate dentist and hygienist); and *(3)* investment of assets (eg, generating dividends from stock or rent from an apartment building). You can achieve your retirement goals through accumulated wealth from earned income as well as passive income from your investment and savings over the years. Therefore, the take-home lesson is that it is important to maximize income, live within your means, and commit to a savings program.

The key to accumulating wealth is to maximize income, live within your means, and commit to a savings program.

Financial independence

Financial independence is the stage at which you no longer have to work because your investment assets yield payouts that support your living expenses. At this stage, many dentists do not actually retire. Instead, they choose to pursue other interests and activities such as joining the Peace Corps or embarking on a whole new career. Others who reach financial independence choose to live in Hawaii to play golf and fish every day. Although it seems odd to consider projected retirement assumptions just as you begin a career, it makes sense to visualize your destination as you are drawing the map that will get you there.

financial independence
The stage at which you no longer have to work because your investment assets yield payouts that support your living expenses.

Considering projected retirement assumptions as you begin your career helps you to visualize your destination and draw the map that will get you there.

One way to determine your retirement income needs is to use a retirement calculator, which you can find on many financial websites. These calculators use the financial model known as a *Monte Carlo simulation*, which mathematically evaluates a retirement plan to determine if it will last a lifetime. Computer software iterations through hundreds or thousands of market-condition scenarios predict the probability that a plan provides retirement income that will outlast the expected lifetime of the retiree. If a plan runs through 10,000 iterations with 10,000 separate scenarios, and it works 8,000 times, that means there is an 80% probability that you won't run out of money. If an 80% probability of success is too risky for you, and you prefer a 90% probability, you can tweak your plan

RETIREMENT CALCULATORS

- T. Rowe Price: www3.troweprice.com/ric/ric/public/ric.do
- Vanguard: personal.vanguard.com/us/planningeducation/retirement/PEdRetInvHowMuchToSaveContent.jsp
- Charles Schwab: www.schwab.com/public/schwab/planning/retirement/retirement_savings_calculator?src=nsw

by adding more money to your hypothetical investment or taking less money out for living expenses.

To test this out for yourself, use one of the online calculators listed at the end of the chapter to assemble a retirement plan that assumes:

- You and your spouse are 30 years and 26 years of age, respectively.
- In aggregate $11,000 is required monthly for retirement living expenses.
- Each respectively earns $150,000 and $50,000 annually.
- Both contribute 23% of their respective annual incomes to a tax-deferred plan.
- Both aggregately contribute $8,000 annually to an individual retirement account.
- The plan is allocated over a life span of time based on expected retirement horizon.
- Both retire upon reaching 65 years of age.
- Both do not receive social security benefits at retirement.
- Both expect to live to 95 years of age.

The simulation should show that both you and your spouse will have sufficient funds to meet income needs upon reaching retirement at age 65.

These online calculators are good tools for estimating the amount you will need to earn in order to meet your current needs as well as your retirement needs. However, it is important not to rely too heavily on these online calculators. According to a recent *Wall Street Journal* article,[1] the simulations found on some websites are not good predictors of true retirement income because they assume that long-term market returns are distributed along a bell-shaped curve and don't take into consideration wide fluctuations like those seen in the 2009 stock market decline.

Geographic goals and objectives

Geographic factors are influential in planning your career strategy. Do you envision tennis and golf, surfing, or skiing; a farm or an urban garden; a dog or a horse; a sensitivity to environmental allergens or an allergy to the in-laws? Your interests, preferences, health issues, and feelings about being close to friends and relatives have a significant impact on where you will choose to live and work. The ease of obtaining state licensure is another consideration, although less so than it was in the past.

Your interests, preferences, health issues, and feelings about being close to friends and relatives have a significant impact on where you will choose to live and work.

Personal considerations

Special interests, personal preferences, and hobbies are factors to consider when choosing a practice location. If you love to surf and enjoy warm climates, then your ideal location is somewhere like Hawaii, California, or Florida. If you're interested in raising a family in a low-key, low cost-of-living region, then maybe your destination is the Midwest.

Personal health issues also may be a priority. For example, for those who are susceptible to seasonal affective disorder, a condition in which a person is adversely affected by a lack of sunshine, locations such as Seattle may be out of the question.

Finally, proximity to family and friends is a major determinant in practice location for many people. Some people like staying on familiar terrain and want to practice in their hometown to be close to immediate family and childhood friends. However, others may have a dysfunctional family situation or the desire to strike out on their own, leading them to choose a location at a distance from their place of origin.

Rocky Mountain High

Richard Nathan, DMD, MS

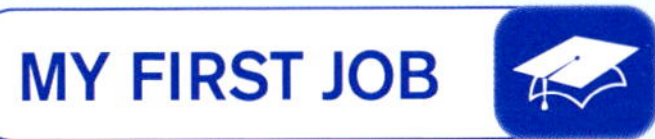

It was the summer of 1975 and I was fresh out of Tufts Dental School when my wife and I moved to Colorado. We had never lived outside of Boston and New York, so we knew life in the Rocky Mountains was going to be a new experience for us, but we were eager to get a taste of western hospitality.

My first job was as a general practice resident (GPR) at Denver General Hospital. Six GPRs rotated through endodontics, periodontics, pedodontics, oral surgery, and restorative dentistry for 2 months alongside an attending specialist. And then, of course, there was the scary rotation–general anesthesia. I mean, what were they thinking? They had dental neophytes put patients to sleep, monitor them during surgery, and then hopefully wake them up. When on call we slept in the hospital. Now, more than 30 years later, if the phone rings in the middle of the night, I still feel that same sense of dread. I would have to drag myself down to the ER half asleep and mentally prepare myself for the knife wound to the face, fractured jaw, or avulsed tooth that would greet me (along with the distinct smell of blood mixed with Jack Daniels). Any patient with trauma above the neck who walked into the ER was ours. I must have placed 3,000 sutures in tongues, lips, cheeks, foreheads, eyelids, and even ears that year.

I got paid $11,500, which was enough to indulge in a new Ford 150 van tricked out with a bed, wood paneling, four speakers, and an eight-track tape deck–what a sweet ride! That van was our home away from home for skiing, fishing, and camping in every corner of the state.

In retrospect, my first job was difficult and yet extremely rewarding. It was an incredible opportunity for growth as a clinician and, most importantly, a means of gaining the confidence I'd need for my future career challenges. The chance to go camping in the Rocky Mountains with my wife wasn't so bad either.

State licensure

In the not-so-distant past, dentists were mandated to pass a clinical test in each state in which they wished to practice. It was a heavy burden on those who moved to a different state midcareer, practiced in multiple states, or were specialists required to take a generalist clinical examination. Fortunately, the dental boards in most states are now more flexible when issuing dental licenses. Historically, Hawaii was one of the most recalcitrant from a licensing perspective, but the state currently accepts the clinical examination of the American Board of Dental Examiners in lieu of its own test. Another attractive state in which to practice, California, does not require any clinical examination, and it will issue a dental license after the completion of an American Dental Association (ADA) Commission on Dental Accreditation (CODA)–approved general practice residency (GPR) or Advanced Education in General Dentistry (AEGD) program. The state of New York issues a dental license based on the successful completion of an accredited dental specialty residency or GPR.

Given the current status of state dental licensure laws, a dentist is now relatively free to choose his or her preferred practice location without onerous constraints.

For initial licensure, state laws permit dental boards to accept the examination results from regional dental clinical testing agencies like the Western Regional Examining Board (WREB) for a period of time (generally 5 years), whether or not the applicant is licensed or has practiced in another state. The only requirement is that the state accepts the results of that regional examination. Given the current status of state dental licensure laws, a dentist is now relatively free to choose his or her preferred practice location without onerous constraints.

licensure by credentials
The process by which a state dental board may grant licensure based on active, continuous practice and licensure in another state as well as successful completion of certain state-specific written ethics and dental law tests.

The requirements to obtain the initial dental license through a clinical test or a residency program must not be confused with licensure by credentials. Licensure by credentials requires active, continuous practice for a specified period of time as well as passing certain state-specific written ethics and dental law tests. Refer to the ADA's website for further information on dental licensure, state dental license recognition, and state membership in the regional clinical testing agencies. Also, check with each state dental board to obtain the most current and specific license requirements, application processes, and fees.

Temporal goals and objectives

Temporal goals and objectives include the pace and time horizon at which to arrive at financial independence. That horizon may very well be the age of 50 years if that's when you expect dentistry to lose its allure and the pursuit of other activities to become more attractive. For others, the allure of dental practice is too compelling to ever retire, and happiness and fulfillment mean going to the office every day to treat patients.

Practice versus leisure time

The pace at which you amble, trot, or run is an important determinant in your career strategy. One way to look at the temporal aspect of pace is to consider your preference in the balance of practice versus leisure time.

Consider the tortoise and the hare. A tortoise takes a slow pace to achieve its goal. If you are a tortoise, you might prefer to spend more time with family and leisure pursuits and may require more time than the hare to attain your financial goals. Most likely the tortoise practices dentistry just enough to meet living expenses and saves at a slower pace; therefore, reaching the finish line of financial independence takes longer. Hopefully the tortoise's family and leisure time is fulfilling.

Are you a tortoise or a hare? A tortoise prefers to spend more time with family and leisure pursuits and may require more time to attain financial goals. A hare practices more days and hours at a faster pace and therefore requires less time to achieve financial independence.

The hare, on the other hand, practices more days and hours than the tortoise at a faster pace and therefore requires less time to achieve financial independence. Of course, in the well-known Aesop fable, the hare eats the carrot as fast as it acquires it and is worse off at the end of the race than the slower-paced tortoise. The wise hare saves as much as possible to avoid this outcome.

DENTAL LICENSURE

- ADA dental licensure: www.ada.org/prof/prac/licensure/information.asp#clinical
- ADA state dental license recognition: www.ada.org/prof/prac/licensure/licensure_recognition.pdf
- ADA state membership in regional clinical testing agencies: www.ada.org/prof/prac/licensure/licensure_regional_testing.pdf

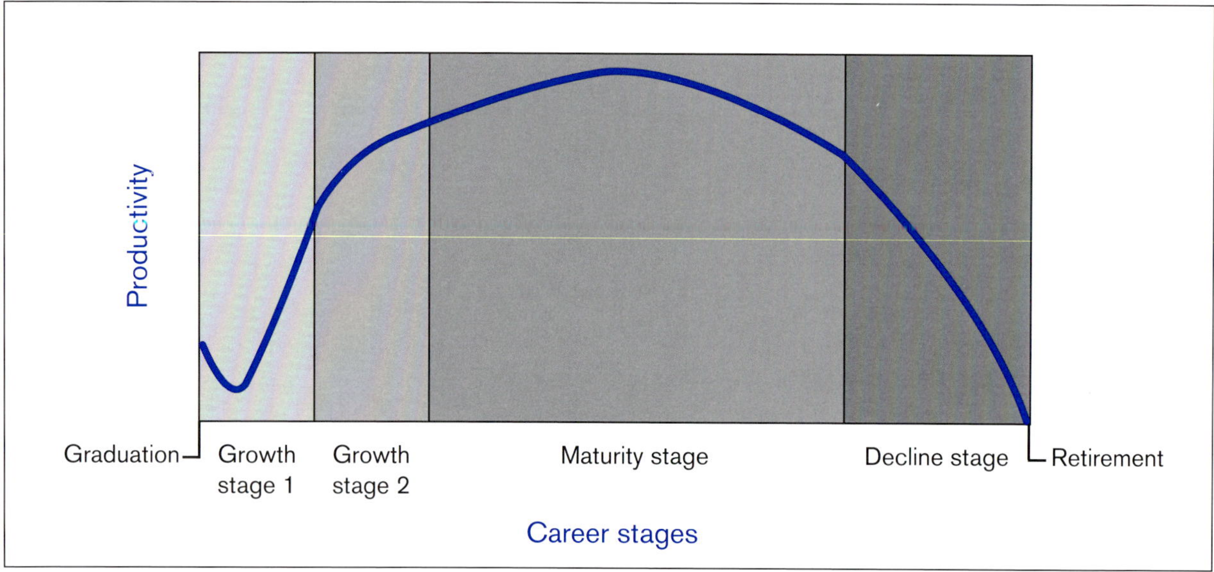

Fig 1-2 Productivity over the course of a career. In the growth stages, the value of money exceeds the value of time. In the maturity stage, the value of time and money is equal. In the decline stage, the value of time exceeds the value of money.

Career stages

Let's look at the time horizon of a practice in terms of the production of income generated over a career from graduation to retirement (Fig 1-2). In the first growth stage, the dentist may earn very little net income because of school, practice, mortgage, and other loan payments and is not yet managerially effective or clinically efficient in providing dental services. During the second growth stage, the dentist may gain enough managerial judgment and clinical efficiency to become productive; therefore, net income increases. During the maturity stage, maximum productivity is usually attained, which means that the practice is relatively stable, debt is paid down, and net income is invested into other assets. At the decline stage–which comes at a different age for each individual–the dentist slows down the pace of practice with the concomitant reduction in productivity and net income.

Money versus time

Money is the currency of professional life, and time is the currency of personal life.

Money is the currency of professional life, and time is the currency of personal life. The dentist has excess time but very little money during the growth stage. So, the value of money exceeds the value of time at this stage. During the maturity stage, one has the luxury of the value of money equaling the value of time. It is during this stage that the previously mentioned tortoise-and-the-hare scenario plays out most strongly, as the dentist finds a balance between the practice, family, and leisure. During the decline stage, the value of time far exceeds the value of money, so the dentist will make a decision about whether he or she would rather spend time on personal leisure or professional fulfillment. Either decision usually results in less money. For example, many senior clinical dental school faculty members teach at a low–or even no–salary. They are driven by the desire for professional fulfillment.

In summary, as you plan your career strategy, remember that the pace at which you earn and save money will determine the time horizon at which you will reach financial independence. Be sure to choose a career path that will allow you to work at the pace you desire and to retire when you are ready to do so.

Internal Resources

We now turn your career strategy planning inward so you can begin to assess your personal resources such as clinical competency, managerial skills, entrepreneurial talent, and financial resources. Other internal resources integral to a practice's strategic plan not addressed in this section include personal ethics, values, and responsibilities.

New York City Tough

Eric Studley, DDS

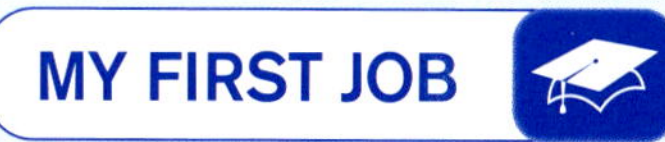

You remember your first job after graduating dental school like you remember your first kiss. For some, it's a good memory, and, for others, it's an eye-opening experience that causes one to question why he or she entered the profession in the first place. The "shelter" of dental school becomes all too apparent once you enter the workforce and are faced with challenges related to ethics, standards of care, and finances.

When I graduated from New York University (NYU) College of Dentistry in 1985, I began my quest to find a job. I bought the Sunday edition of *The New York Times* and searched the classified ads under the letter *D* and the professional practices under the "Business Opportunities" section. There was no email or fax at the time, so I called around that Monday to arrange for potential interviews.

My first interview was with a union dental clinic above a bank in an outlying borough of New York City. It was my first interview, and I didn't know what questions to ask or what to expect for compensation. The interview consisted of them asking me when I could start working and what days I could work, and my compensation was set at 30% of production with a guarantee of $200 a day. I was offered 3 days a week and was ecstatic that I had a job. I needed to work 6 days a week to cover my expenses, so I set out to look for a second job.

My second interview was at a shopping mall practice with hours of operation until 9 pm. I filled some additional days and hours there. The interview focused on the amount of patients I could treat in a day and the necessity of working evenings and Saturdays. The compensation was set at 35% of production with no minimum guarantee per day. Once again, I was elated to find any employment and accepted the position.

The union dental clinic was, to say the least, surprising. I learned on the first day of work that the office didn't have an autoclave, an amalgamator, or even an automatic x-ray developer. There were only one or two high-speed drills that worked. I had to wait to use one if the owner was using it at that time. Dental materials were scarce and inadequate at best. However, I genuinely liked the two owners of the practice. I stayed until I was offered a full-time position at the second job a couple of months later.

That second job was mostly an insurance dental practice where high volume, low fees, and fast pace with no breaks were the expectation. Fortunately, the facility and equipment were new. I was the only dentist working with the two owners at first, but the practice grew rapidly, and eventually they hired multiple dentists and specialists. The office was open 7 days a week, and after accepting the full-time position, I was told that working Sundays was required if I wanted to keep the other days. I relented because I had left my first job and couldn't afford to lose this one. I worked more than 60 hours a week and treated a high volume of patients per day. I constantly argued with the employers because they always paid less than what was expected for unscrupulous reasons. Throughout my tenure I was treated unprofessionally, unethically, and, at times, disrespectfully. Nevertheless, I stayed for nearly 2 years because I didn't want to leave for another job, knowing that at some point I wanted to purchase my own practice. So I changed my attitude and looked at the situation as a phenomenal learning experience. I acquired a tremendous amount of business knowledge on how to run a practice, manage employees, and build a practice. I used the negative experience to grow my own practice with a positive attitude.

Look at your first job as a growth experience, whether it's positive or negative. It takes 4 years to graduate from dental school, so don't give up easily on your vision and aspirations. Hold on to your ethical standard and your level of patient care. Once your vision becomes a reality, you will know why you entered the profession.

Clinical competency

Clinical competency is an internal resource that the dental school and state dental board deem each licensee to possess to be competent enough to practice dentistry. However, when you are ready to start practicing, you must make a realistic assessment of your skills to determine the level at which you will be able to practice efficiently and with a high degree of quality. A realistic self-assessment may lead you to begin practicing dentistry as an employee for a community clinic, where the process allows room to acquire increased competency and speed. On the other end of the spectrum, if your clinical skills are manifestly evident, you may opt for the immediate purchase of an upper eastside Manhattan cosmetic and spa dental practice.

clinical competency
An internal resource that the dental school and state dental board deem each licensee to possess to be able to practice dentistry. The *degree* of clinical competency you possess should play a role in your career strategy.

Managerial skills

Some qualities of a good manager include:

- High energy level
- Objectivity
- Ability to work under stress and uncertainty
- Good interpersonal skills
- Leadership qualities
- Cognizance of the political and cultural environment
- Effective problem-solving abilities, such as fact finding, organizing, planning, and decision making
- Ability to communicate verbally and nonverbally with clarity and persuasiveness

If you weren't born with the skills you need to be an effective manager, consider enrolling in managerial and communication courses offered through a local or online community college or continuing education institution.

If you are unsure whether you possess these qualities, a self-assessment test such as the one provided on the Humanlinks website may be helpful. If the self-assessment shows that you are not currently well suited to being a manager, do not despair. Managerial skills can be developed–consider enrolling in managerial and communication courses offered through a local or online community college or continuing education institution.

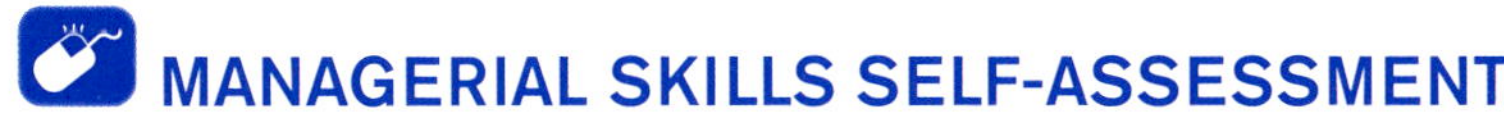

- www.humanlinks.com/check.htm

Entrepreneurial skills

Having an entrepreneurial spirit is a significant advantage for dentists, particularly those who plan to enter private practice.

Your entrepreneurial skill level will also influence your career strategy. Dentists require some level of expertise as an entrepreneur because the majority of them will enter private practice. Successful entrepreneurs generally are:

- Self-confident
- Hard working
- Flexible
- Driven
- Committed
- Visionary
- Idealistic
- Innovative
- Multitalented
- Goal oriented
- Risk tolerant
- Creative
- Dedicated
- Passionate
- Task oriented
- Stubborn
- Self-motivated
- Stress tolerant
- Perfectionistic

There are some online assessment tests you can take to determine whether or not you have what it takes to be an entrepreneur.

Financial resources

Financial resources vary widely among graduates of dental school. Some have a huge amount of accrued educational debt that may take 8 to 14 years to repay. Others have parents who paid for much of their education, and a very small number are members of a wealthy family and have nothing to pay back. Each dentist must assess his or her current personal financial position–no matter how painful–to determine an individual career strategy.

It is important to take an honest look at your current personal financial position as you determine your career strategy.

Two essential financial tools used to assess financial position include the income statement and the net worth statement (ie, the balance sheet). Preparing these statements helps you understand your strengths and weaknesses as you plan an effective business strategy and is a required step in applying for any loan or line of credit. Be sure to prepare separate personal and business financial statements.

Preparing income and net worth statements helps you understand your strengths and weaknesses as you plan an effective business strategy and gives you a head start in applying for a loan or line of credit.

ENTREPRENEURIAL SKILLS SELF-ASSESSMENT

- Brigham Young University Marriott School Center for Entrepreneurship & Technology: marriottschool.byu.edu/cfe/startingout/test.cfm
- US Small Business Administration: web.sba.gov/sbtn/sbat/index.cfm?Tool=4

Flexibility and Freedom

Francis Serio, DMD, MS, MBA

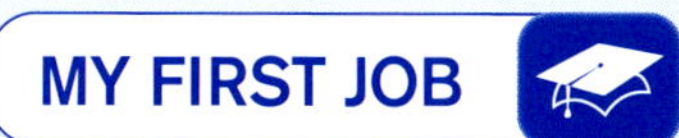

One of the most important advantages I gave myself as an undergraduate in private college and as a dental student was to carefully manage my finances. The result was that I had only $5,000 in total student loans upon finishing dental school. Many of my friends were at least $75,000 in debt, even in 1980. I managed to keep my debt small by banking 90% of everything I earned since I was young and keeping my personal expenses to a minimum throughout school. The pit I lived in while in dental school horrified my mother, but by watching everything I spent, I managed to get by without financial aid until my last year of dental school. Of course, having supportive and generous parents helped a lot.

After my GPR, I looked at several private practice opportunities. During that search, I came across an advertisement for a job at the University of Maryland. Teaching always interested me, so I decided to apply for the position. That was the beginning of what has been a rewarding 28-year academic career. I could afford to take a job that paid only $26,500 because my debt obligation was so minimal–just a small student loan payment and a note for my first car, a Chevrolet Chevette (check the history books). At Maryland I taught four-handed dentistry, covered the dental auxiliary utilization (DAU) clinic, and started an honors program based on concepts I learned during my residency. After 3 years of teaching and maintaining a private practice, I enrolled in a periodontic specialty program that launched me into the next phase of my career.

Although it may be necessary to incur debt to meet your goals, remember that minimizing your debt translates into maximum flexibility and freedom of choice.

Income statement

The income statement lists gross revenue and expenses over a period of time, usually a calendar year. The arithmetic difference between revenue and expenses directly related to operating a dental practice is operating income. When you subtract other factors such as interest, tax, depreciation, and amortization from operating income, you get net income.

Of course, *positive operating income* means the practice earns more than it spends, and the surplus is available for personal use and investment. A *negative operating income* (ie, loss) means that the practice must borrow from a line of credit to stay afloat. This situation of negative operating in-

income statement
Lists gross revenue and expenses over a period of time, usually a calendar year.

operating income
Revenue minus expenses directly related to operating the business.

net income
Operating income minus interest, tax, depreciation, amortization, and any other nonoperating business expenses.

come cannot go on indefinitely: The practice must generate more revenue, cut expenses, do both, or go out of business. There are a number of online resources that can assist you with these calculations.

Net worth statement

net worth statement *or* balance sheet
Document presenting your assets minus your liabilities at one given point in time.

The net worth statement, or balance sheet, calculates your net worth or asset value at one given point in time. This statement can be generated at any time; however, once a year is sufficient for many individuals of modest wealth.

Net worth is determined by the algebraic equation

$$\text{Net worth} = \text{Assets} - \text{Liabilities}$$

or any other algebraic permutation, such as

$$\text{Assets} = \text{Liabilities} + \text{Net worth.}$$

A *positive net worth* means there are more assets than liabilities. For the accounting geeks among dentists, other information can be gleaned from a net worth statement, such as liquidity, profitability, and financial leverage, that takes into consideration current and long-term assets and liabilities, allocation, and the use of debt. High financial leverage–using debt (ie, loans) with the assumption that the money borrowed will generate substantially more revenue–is expected in startup and purchased dental practices.

high financial leverage
Using debt (ie, loans) with the assumption that the money borrowed will generate substantially more revenue in the future—usually a necessary measure when starting up or purchasing a practice.

The net worth statement should be updated annually to determine the progress of your business strategy. There are a number of online resources that can assist with net worth calculations.

External Environment

The external environment defines the playing field in which you can create your career strategy. Clearly answering the following questions will help you to realistically formulate your goals and objectives within the boundaries of your environment:

- What is the competitive market of dentists in the chosen location?
- What is the patient demographic of this location?
- Is the current macroeconomic climate and microeconomic financial market favorable for a dental loan?

- Is there a qualified pool of dental staff readily available?
- What percentage of the potential patient population has dental insurance?
- Does managed care affect competition?
- What is the state income tax? Is it low like Nevada's or sky-high like New Jersey's?

Competition

As is discussed in the section on career paths later in this chapter, the majority of dentists in the US choose a career in private practice, so competition is a critical factor when evaluating your external environment. Based on the US Census Bureau's population estimates for 2009,[2] there are 1,691 patients for every dentist. This ratio serves as a benchmark for competitive market research.

It is relatively easy to estimate the number of practicing dentists in a given geographic area. One method is to enter *dentists* and the name of the city in which you plan to practice into an online search engine, which will bring up a number of website references with lists of dentists located in your city. Other resources include the online directories of professional organizations such as the ADA or your state or local dental association. Keep in mind that dentist population data are inflated in areas with dental schools or large retirement communities because they include dental school faculty and licensed but nonpracticing dentists. Once you've determined approximately how many dentists are practicing in your location, estimate the patient population. There are a number of online resources that provide population estimates.

PROFIT VERSUS LOSS CALCULATIONS

- Yahoo! Finance: finance.yahoo.com/calculator/banking-budgeting/bud-09
- Bankrate: www.bankrate.com/brm/calc/Worksheet.asp

NET WORTH CALCULATIONS

- CNN Money: cgi.money.cnn.com/tools/networth/networth.html
- Yahoo! Finance: finance.yahoo.com/calculator/career-work/bud-07
- Bankrate: www.bankrate.com/brm/calculators/personalfinance/net_worth_calculator.asp

DIRECTORY OF DENTAL PROFESSIONALS

- American Dental Association: www.ada.org/members/directory/index.asp

For illustration, let's say the town you are planning to practice in–we'll call it Anytown–has approximately 107 dentists and a population of 122,000. Therefore, the dentist-to-population ratio is 1:1,140. This ratio is significantly lower than the 1:1,691 ratio for the entire United States; therefore, the competitive environment for patients in Anytown is higher than the average for the United States.

Consumer market

The consumer market, or the patient pool, is another critical external environment factor. The same online resources that provide population estimates can also be searched for patient demographic data such as income, education, race, age, and family size. Imagine that the US Census Bureau shows that in Anytown the median household income is $55,597 and the household size is 2.74 persons. Note that the median income (where one half of the incomes are above and one half are below) is a better figure to use than the mean income (ie, arithmetic average) because it is less sensitive to distortion caused by extremes. Table 1-1 compares the demographic parameters between Anytown and the entire state. In this hypothetical situation, the median household income of Anytown is greater than that of the state, although it has fewer persons per household. Therefore, Anytown's potential patient population makes it an appealing choice for practice location even though the population-to-dentist ratio is low.

median income
Middle point of the range of incomes in an area, with half of residents having incomes above the median, and the other half having incomes below the median. This figure is less sensitive to distortion caused by extremes than is mean income.

mean income
Arithmetic average of incomes in an area.

Financial market

The financial market determines the availability of capital to borrow to meet your goals and objectives. Capital obtained from a loan is needed to finance, for example, postdoctoral study, practice startup or purchase, a car to drive to the new job, or a wedding.

At the time this chapter was written in March 2009, the financial market was experiencing a historic and significant downturn. The Dow Jones Industrial Average lost nearly 50% of its capitalization from March 2008 to March 2009[3]; the unemployment rate soared to 8%[4]; the financial industry, including major commercial banks, investment banks, and insurers, received federal bailout money; and the automobile industry required

POPULATION ESTIMATES/DEMOGRAPHICS

- US Census Bureau: quickfacts.census.gov/qfd/states
- City-Data: www.city-data.com

Table 1-1 Demographics of a hypothetical consumer market

Demographic	Anytown	State
Total population	122,204	36.5 million
Median household income	$55,597	$49,894
Persons per household	2.74	2.87
Ethnicity		
Caucasian	70.7%	59.5%
Hispanic	21.8%	32.4%
Other	7.5%	8.1%

government intervention to stave off bankruptcy. Fortunately, however, in 2009, banks and financial institutions continued to lend money to dentists for practice purchase and startups despite the dismal economic environment:

- Bank of America was writing dental practice loans from $100,000 to $5 million with 100% financing at a fixed rate for up to 15 years with deferred, graduated, and interest-only repayment options.[5] Working capital could be added, and the practice and a real estate loan could be combined.
- Matsco, a division of Wells Fargo Bank, was touting its competitive, fixed-rate dental practice loan with preferred interest rates and other benefits for ADA members. Its loans were financed up to 100% with terms to fit a fledgling budget.[6] It offered deferred payment programs for practice purchase loans and a graduated payment program for practice startup loans. Matsco also offered a working capital line of credit.
- Henry Schein was prequalifying loans for $400,000 by application-only status and a same-day approval process.[7] The company wrote loans for leasehold improvement, working capital, or construction financing. Henry Schein would customize a loan repayment schedule to fit cash

LENDING AGENCIES

- Bank of America: www.bankofamerica.com/vehicle_and_personal_loans/index.cfm?template=practice_sales_and_purchases
- Matsco: www.matsco.com/dentists/practice-financing-programs/practice-start-up-financing.htm
- Henry Schein: www.henryschein.com/us-en/dental/services/Financial/PracticeStartup.aspx
- GE Healthcare Financial Services: www.gehealthcarefinance.com/OurSolutions/LandingPages/GE_Practiceacquisition.aspx

flow and financial requirements and work with the dentist to create a business plan, budget, and cash flow statement.

- GE Healthcare Financial Services, a company that specializes in practice acquisition finance, was working with dentists to evaluate their financial viability and opportunity. GE broke down its loan process into five steps[8]: *(1)* Apply and qualify for the loan, *(2)* evaluate the practice, *(3)* prepare the loan terms, *(4)* finalize the contract, and *(5)* accept terms and sign loan-closing documents.

The March 2009 issue of *TIME* magazine featured an article[9] explaining that dentists were faring financially well during the 2009 recession because:

- Patients were visiting the dentist to take advantage of their insurance benefits
- Dental disease worsens over time
- Deferred dental treatment leads to more expensive treatment later
- Patients prefer to spend their money on dental care rather than put that money into a falling stock market

The business of dentistry is relatively immune to the economic shocks and downturns that face other professions and industries.

This shows that we are truly fortunate to have chosen dentistry as a career because the business of dentistry is relatively immune to the economic shocks and downturns that face other professions and industries.

Labor market

The ready availability of qualified labor is important to consider when formulating a career strategy. Is there a pool of dental assistants and dental hygienists in the area? Are a large number of other recent graduates looking for the same associate dentist job? If you want to be a military or academic dentist, how many other qualified dentists are competing for the same position or appointment?

Labor information can be obtained from the website of the US Bureau of Labor Statistics. Information is posted on the average wage and number of workers in different job categories. Enter the phrase *labor market statistics* and the name of your state into a search engine to find links to state-specific and county-specific labor data.

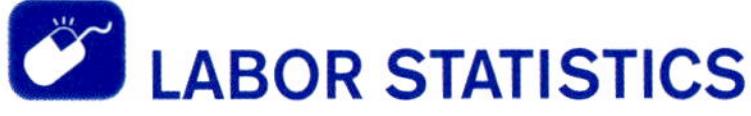

LABOR STATISTICS

- US Bureau of Labor Statistics: www.bls.gov/

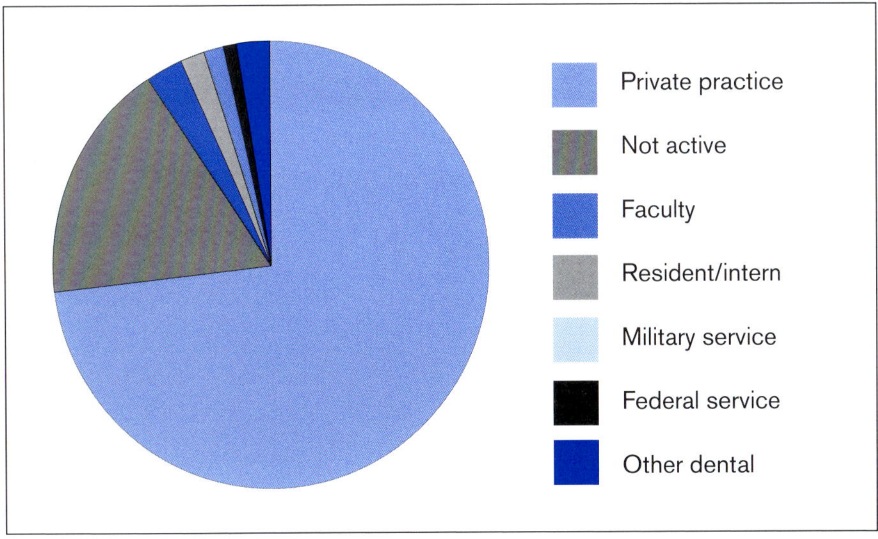

Fig 1-3 Distribution of dentists in various career categories in 2003.

Government regulation

At every level of regulation (ie, federal, state, and local), there are taxes: income, employment, sales, personal property, inheritance (death), and excise. Every level also requires licensure, such as the federal Drug Enforcement Agency license to prescribe controlled substances; the state dental board license to practice dentistry; and the city and county business license to open your office. Federal and state employment laws impact a dentist whether he or she is the employer or the employee. The dental office is required to comply with certain health, safety, and privacy regulations such as the Occupational Safety and Health Administration (OSHA) and the Health Information Portability and Accountability Act (HIPAA).

Career Paths

Now that you have examined and assessed your goals and objectives as well as your internal resources and the external environment, it is time to use that information to evaluate your potential career paths.

For 72.6% of dentists in the United States, a career path leads to private practice in some form[10] (Fig 1-3). Other career paths include military and federal service as well as academic faculty appointments. Some dental graduates postpone their career decisions to pursue postdoctorate education as graduate students, interns, or residents.

The University of North Carolina School of Dentistry website is the source of much of the information in this chapter and provides an excellent overview of options for your career path. The Student Doctor Network's online dental forums offer some helpful information as well.

Military Service Dentistry

Practicing dentistry in a branch of the armed forces is an attractive career option. Military dentists usually work in a group practice setting, and the camaraderie can be intoxicating. Most military dentists treat 40 to 80 patients per week.

Some advantages of military service include a secure and reasonable salary with merit-based pay increases, career longevity, and promotions with increased responsibility. A benefits package may include free medical care and a discounted health care plan for the family, disability benefits, and retirement pay with benefits. A military dentist is also immediately eligible for retirement pay and benefits after 20 years of active duty service. The military provides the opportunity for continuing education with possible reimbursement for registration fees, travel, and lodging expenses for approved classes. Dentists enter the military as uniformed officers, and the active duty military dental officer is eligible for 30 days of paid vacation and 11 paid holidays each year.

In 2009, depending on attained rank and service time, the base monthly compensation ranged from $2,655 per month (officer 1 rank with less than 2 years of service) to $18,061 per month (officer 10 rank with more than 38 years of service).[11] Base compensation rates do not include additional allowances, such as those for subsistence, housing, variable special pay, and dental additional special pay. A hypothetical example of the annual compensation for an unmarried army captain with the rank of officer 3 and less than 3 years of service is shown in Table 1-2. The Defense Finance and Accounting Service website provides the basic pay and allowance charts that apply to each branch of the armed services.

CAREER OPTIONS

- University of North Carolina School of Dentistry: www.dent.unc.edu/careers/career_options/CareersIndex2.cfm
- Student Doctor Network's dental forums: forums.studentdoctor.net/forumdisplay.php?f=55

Table 1-2 Hypothetical breakdown of annual military compensation*

Type	Amount (US $)
Base pay	48,161
Basic allowance for subsistence	2,676
Average basic allowance for housing	12,809
Tax benefit†	6,293
Variable special pay	3,000
Dental additional special pay	10,000
Total annual compensation	**82,939**

*Data from Defense Finance and Accounting Service.[11]

†Basic allowance for subsistence and basic allowance for housing are exempt from federal/state taxes and excluded from social security taxes.

Of course, there are some disadvantages to being a dentist in the military. First and foremost, you may be assigned to combat duty and separated from family for a long period of time. Even if you are not deployed, relocation to different station bases occurs every 3 to 5 years. The overall salary is less than that earned in full-time private practice. A superior officer may evaluate your clinical performance, and that rating impacts potential merit bonuses and promotions. As a junior officer, the types of clinical procedures performed may be limited to simple procedures.

A military career fits the nonentrepreneurial, regimented type of person with a desire for travel and camaraderie.

Consider your career strategy and how military dentistry does or does not fit your puzzle pieces. A military career fits the nonentrepreneurial, regimented type of person with a desire for travel and camaraderie. To find out more about opportunities with specific branches of the military, see their websites.

MILITARY COMPENSATION

- Defense Finance and Accounting Service: www.dfas.mil/militarypay/militarypaytables.html

MILITARY DENTAL CAREER OPTIONS

- Air Force: www.airforce.com/opportunities/healthcare/careers/dentistry/
- Army: www.goarmy.com/amedd/dental/corps_benefits.jsp
- Navy: www.navy.com/careers/healthcare/dentist/

Tropical Breeze

Michael Okuji, DDS, MPH, MBA

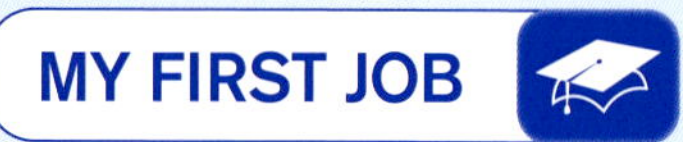

I found my first job after a federal budget cut axed my research fellowship. Without money to live on and no dental school loan reprieve, my plan for a biochemistry PhD came to an abrupt end. That summer I had plenty of time on my hands and no job prospects at all. One day, out of sheer boredom, I accompanied a classmate to his job interview for a position as a public health dentist. While I was waiting for my friend to complete his interview, another recruiter began talking to me and ended up offering me a job as a public health dentist in Guam. I had never given a thought to public health dentistry and couldn't locate Guam on a map. I was young and single with no money in the bank, so I accepted on the spot and found myself on a plane to Guam within the month. The job came with a livable wage, insurance, housing, and a round-trip flight back home every year.

Guam is an island of Micronesia in the North Pacific Ocean, about three-quarters of the way from Hawaii to Indonesia. I landed there with two other recent graduates. We lived in Quonset huts and shared duties at two public health clinics. Schoolchildren were bussed to the main clinic every morning. Two of us worked with eight other dentists who were trained in the Philippines and acted as expanded-duty assistants. We would first anesthetize a row of children, then return to the first and prep each one. The assistants placed the restorations. Those assistants had their hands full keeping us new guys out of trouble. Our efficiency increased every day, and I was pretty proficient in restorations and extractions when I returned home.

The 5-mile-wide island enjoyed tropical weather and crystal clear blue water, and we had plenty of free time to water-ski, sail, and scuba. Dentistry took me to the islands of Saipan, Yap, Pohnpei, Palau, and Truk. New and exotic experiences were found around every coconut tree. It was a heck of an adventure for a kid who had never traveled beyond Southern California.

Given the circumstances of my very first job, I was the Prince of Serendipity if not Sagacity. I didn't hesitate for a second to grasp good fortune as it passed. In hindsight, it all worked out for the best. I returned home after 2 years and started my practice from scratch. I'm much happier with my gregarious private practice than I ever would have been working on a solitary bench in a research laboratory.

Federal Service Dentistry

Dentistry in the federal service is a multifaceted career path. Clinical career opportunities include the National Health Service Corps (NHSC), Indian Health Service (IHS), US Coast Guard, and the Federal Bureau of Prisons. All are administered by the US Public Health Service (USPHS) Commissioned Corps under the Department of Health and Human Services.

US Public Health Service Commissioned Corps

The USPHS commissions approximately 6,000 health professionals to serve federal government agencies and programs.[12] The advantage of service as a uniformed dental officer in the Commissioned Corps is that the dentist can focus on clinical practice without the demands of starting and maintaining a dental practice. Another benefit is the leadership opportunities not found in private practice. Although the USPHS is not a military branch, the USPHS Commissioned Corps is one of seven uniformed services of the US government.[13]

A uniformed dental officer in the Commissioned Corps can focus on clinical practice without the demands of starting and maintaining a dental practice.

In 2009, a USPHS dentist who agreed to serve at least 4 years was eligible for a $60,000 sign-up bonus.[13] The annual compensation for a dentist employed with the USPHS is calculated on the same basis as for a military dentist, and USPHS employees share benefits similar to those in the military. Officers receive 30 paid vacation days and 10 paid federal holidays per year and may take sick leave as needed.[13] Comprehensive health care for employees and their families is provided. USPHS provides officers with malpractice liability that is covered by the Federal Tort Claims Act at no cost to the employee, and employees also benefit from both noncontributory and contributory retirement plans.[13]

For more information on dental career opportunities in the USPHS Commissioned Corps, see their website.

National Health Service Corps

The NHSC is a very attractive career path for a dentist. The NHSC offers a dental school loan repayment program, a competitive starting salary, and the opportunity to hone dental expertise, sharpen dental judgment, increase efficiency, and develop managerial skills. You can contact the NHSC as early as your first year of dental school.

The NHSC offers a dental school loan repayment program, a competitive starting salary, and the opportunity to hone dental expertise, sharpen dental judgment, increase efficiency, and develop managerial skills.

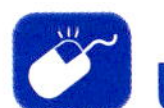

US PUBLIC HEALTH SERVICE COMMISSIONED CORPS

- Dentist page: www.usphs.gov/profession/dentist/default.aspx

Loan repayment program

A major benefit is the NHSC loan repayment program, which in 2009 was repaying up to $50,000 in loans in exchange for a 2-year contract for NHSC service. After graduation, the dentist practices in an NHSC-approved community site and is paid a competitive salary with benefits.

Employment contracts

NHSC employment contract negotiations are solely the responsibility of the dentist. Compensation packages are negotiated directly between the dentist and the NHSC-approved community site. Note that a community clinic cannot guarantee that its employee will receive an NHSC loan repayment contract award; therefore, NHSC loan repayments must not be part of employment and salary negotiations between dentist and community clinic. The terms of employment are typically stipulated in a written employment contract. Terms of the contract should be carefully reviewed and fully understood before the contract is signed. Dentists may want to seek legal guidance from private counsel before entering into any employment contract.

Compensation

According to the author's personal communication with directors of community clinics that sponsor NHSC dentists, an NHSC dentist is compensated from $400 to $600 per 8-hour day. The current NHSC loan repayment agreement states that the dentist must work full time for at least 2 years. *Full time* is defined as 40 hours per week for at least 45 weeks annually.[14] This translates to an annual gross compensation range from $90,000 to $135,000. This is an excellent starting salary for any dental graduate.

Serving public need

The NHSC dentist delivers health care to the millions of adults and children who live in areas nearly devoid of health care professionals.

NHSC offers dentists the opportunity to live and work in communities around the country in urban, rural, or frontier areas. NHSC delivers primary health care service to designated underserved areas at NHSC-approved community sites. The NHSC dentist delivers health care to the millions of adults and children who live in areas nearly devoid of health care professionals. Nearly 4,000 NHSC clinicians serve approximately 4 million underserved Americans.[15]

Working together with community leaders, health administrators, educators, and local government, the NHSC is an integral part of an extraordinary group of dedicated and highly skilled health professionals who are committed to bringing quality health care to the nation's areas of greatest need. Dentists, in conjunction with other members of the primary health care team, make oral health an integral part of total health care. In addition to prevention and early detection of gum disease, tooth loss, and oral cancer, the NHSC dentist's duties include diagnosis of oral conditions, development of treatment plans, administration of anesthetics, treatment of diseased gums, and instruction on brushing, flossing, and diet.

The dental loan repayment program, compensation, clinical skills growth, and fulfillment offered by this career option are compelling reasons to consider the NHSC for your first job. For more information, visit the NHSC website.

Indian Health Services

The IHS addresses the needs of more than 1.6 million American Indians and Alaska Natives.[13] Although some clinic locations are remote, employees work in a modern environment, equipped as well as–or better than–some private practices. In addition to clinical practice, many IHS dentists participate in the development and implementation of community-based prevention programs. IHS dental programs offer opportunities in more than 230 hospitals and clinics across 35 states.[13] The IHS currently employs approximately 1,800 dentists, hygienists, and assistants.[13] The organization recruits dentists who enjoy the adventure of living and practicing in a wide range of geographic locations. The federal personnel system also removes many of the mobility barriers imposed by state licensing requirements. For more information about dental careers in the IHS, visit their website.

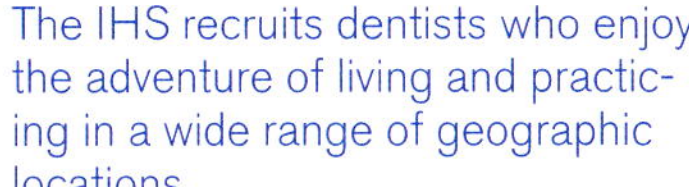
The IHS recruits dentists who enjoy the adventure of living and practicing in a wide range of geographic locations.

US Coast Guard

The US Coast Guard has 58 dentists in 30 clinics located mainly along the Atlantic, Gulf of Mexico, and Pacific coasts, including Alaska, Hawaii, and Puerto Rico.[16] Most Coast Guard clinics are small, and dental officers provide a full range of services, including operative, endodontic, peri-

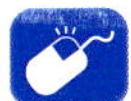

NATIONAL HEALTH SERVICE CORPS

- Official website: nhsc.bhpr.hrsa.gov/

INDIAN HEALTH SERVICES

- Dentist page: www.dentist.ihs.gov/

odontic, oral surgery, prosthodontic, and limited orthodontic procedures. Most patients are active-duty Coast Guard or other military service members. The clinics do not normally provide dental care for geriatric and pediatric patients. The Coast Guard has the highest dentist retention rate of all the uniformed services.[16]

The Coast Guard has the highest dentist retention rate of all the uniformed services.

Federal Bureau of Prisons

The Federal Bureau of Prisons provides dental services in 114 correctional institutions across the country.[17] This unique patient population presents interesting challenges. The patients have different prison security levels, cultural backgrounds, and geographic origins, and they often present with unusual oral pathologies and complex treatment plans.

The dentist interacts with his or her professional colleagues in medicine, psychology, and other disciplines to optimize the delivery of dental care. As with the military and IHS, the Bureau of Prisons offers geographic mobility. Dentists may transfer to different locations throughout the United States, and there are opportunities to choose metropolitan areas such as New York City or Los Angeles, a midsized town, or a rural community. A mentoring program with a regional dental consultant eases the transition to prison health care. The keen camaraderie of these dentists combined with the Bureau's philosophy of the "Bureau family" affords them a sense of belonging and fosters development of lifelong friendships.[17]

The keen camaraderie of Prison Bureau dentists combined with the philosophy of the "Bureau family" affords them a sense of belonging and fosters development of lifelong friendships.

Dental School Faculty

You may choose to pursue a faculty position at one of the 56 dental schools in the United States and Puerto Rico or at a university-based graduate program. Open positions are usually posted online. The number of newly created dental schools is rising following a period of closures; however, there is a scarcity of open faculty positions relative to the number of students graduating from dental school annually.[18]

Keep in mind that a career in academe can expand beyond the positions of department chair and dental school dean. Historically, academic dentists have provided leadership outside of the dental school environment as president of university academic senates, executive vice chancellor of university campuses, provost of university systems, and chancellors and presidents of major universities. Academic dentists have occupied these university-wide positions at the University of California at Los Angeles

Chicago Serendipity

Frank Licari, DDS, MPH, MBA

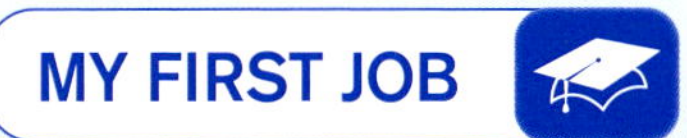

My specific goal after graduation from dental school in 1986 was to own a dental practice. I reviewed all the dental practices for sale in the Chicago area and decided to purchase an office in a far western suburb. However, during negotiation the deal fell through at the last moment, and I was unable to purchase the practice.

A few days later, when I was visiting some friends at the University of Illinois at Chicago College of Dentistry, I ran into the dean. He asked me where I was practicing, and I told him about the failed practice purchase deal. Right on the spot he offered me a job taking radiographs in the oral radiology department. I accepted the offer immediately because I wasn't working anywhere else. That job led to another job treating emergency and challenging patients, which led to another job treating hospital and compromised patients, which led to a teaching appointment that marked the beginning of my 21 years in academic dentistry.

I did open my own dental practice a year after starting my first dental job and practiced for 12 years. But, it was that first job that had the most influence on my career and life.

and San Francisco, Michigan State University, the University of Connecticut, and Tufts University.

Responsibilities

Dental school faculty engage in four major activities: teaching, research, service, and patient care. Significant, high-quality activity is expected in each area to merit promotion and tenure.

- *Teaching* comprises 40% to 55% of faculty time, which can include classroom lecture, treatment supervision, postdoctoral mentoring, and resident training. The departmental chair evaluates the effectiveness of the faculty's teaching performance.
- *Research* is the mission of a major university and an absolute requirement for tenure. The pressure to "publish or perish" continues unabated. The pursuit and acquisition of steady research grant funding is expected to support the research effort.

- *Service* to the community and profession may encompass involvement in committees and organizational activities on and off campus.[18] Intramural activities include participation and leadership on committees and projects at the dental school and university. Extramural participation in local and national dental organizations, journal review boards, and community projects is expected, as is consultation to government or private health-related agencies.
- *Patient care* is provided through the faculty practice. This enables the faculty to maintain and sharpen clinical skills, refine new treatment modalities, and provide a model for dental students and residents. Dentists adept at implant procedures are now the featured dentists in a faculty practice.

Salary

Faculty practice generates income for the practitioner and the school, and it is not unusual for certain academic dentists to earn $300,000 or more based on basic salary, research grants, and practice income. However, in general, the chasm between dental school faculty salary and private practice income continues to grow. Between 1990 and 2000 the base annual salary of full-time dental faculty increased 25% to 30%.[19] During those same 10 years the net income of a full-time solo private practice dentist increased 78%.[19] In 1999 the average income of a full-time solo private practice dentist was $168,000, whereas the average base salary of a full-time clinical faculty with the rank of professor was $103,100.[19] This difference in compensation is magnified when one considers the significant amount of time it takes to reach the rank of full professor compared with the short time it takes to reach the average salary of a private-practice dentist. The annual compensation without outside income from research grants or faculty practice is $80,400 for a full-time clinical associate professor and $67,550 for a full-time assistant professor. The demonstrated difference in salary is staggering, with dentists in private practice earning 109% to 149% of the income earned by dental faculty.[19]

Dental faculty positions are difficult to come by and do not pay as well as a career in private practice. However, you may possess the skill set and inclination to have a successful and rewarding career in dental academics.

But again, consider your particular career goals and objectives. Perhaps the idea of performing research, teaching, and providing service to the community are more appealing to you than making more money in private practice; you may even have the assertiveness, innovation, and unique skill set required to rise to the highest echelon of administration and compensation.

Table 1-3 Immediate career plans after dental school: 2004 graduates*

Immediate plans	Graduates (%)
Private practice	50.4
Solo	4.1
Partnership/group	6.0
Associate/employed	40.3
Advanced education	38.6
Dental school faculty	0.5
Government service	7.5
Undecided	2.9

*Data from American Dental Association Council on Dental Practice.[20]

Private Practice

Private practice, in its many forms, is the primary occupation of dentists. In fact, in 2003, 72.6% of all dentists were in private practice, earning an average annual salary of $218,990.[10,21] A dentist in private practice may be a nonowner associate dentist, an owner dentist who starts a practice from scratch, or an owner dentist who purchases all or part of an existing dental practice. A private practice may be set up as a solo practice, partnership, solo group practice, integrated small or large group practice, single or multispecialty group practice, and multilocation group practice, all of which can adopt the business format of the employee, sole proprietor, or professional corporation. Approximately 50% of new dentists go directly into private practice, with the majority entering as nonowner associates (Table 1-3).

Approximately 50% of new dentists go directly into private practice, with the majority entering as nonowner associates.

Associate (nonowner) dentist

A nonowner dentist in private practice is an employee or independent contractor who is usually called an associate. In private practice, 85.6% of all dentists are sole proprietors,[22] and many hire associates. The primary reason a sole proprietor dentist hires an associate is to allow the owner to work fewer hours (Box 1-1). An advantage to being an associate in a sole proprietorship practice is that a seasoned owner can act as a mentor, teaching the associate the art and business of dentistry. In addition, there is only one boss to report to in the sole proprietorship practice. The associate enjoys the benefit of immediate income and minimal man-

associate
A nonowner dentist in private practice who works as an employee or independent contractor.

Box 1-1 Top 5 reasons dentists hire associate dentists*

1. Work fewer hours
2. Increase patient load of practice
3. Train someone to take over practice
4. Looking toward retirement
5. Current patient load is greater than the dentist can treat alone

*Based on data from Halley et al.[23]

Table 1-4 American Dental Association compensation data for new nonowner dentists*

Compensation arrangement	Respondents (%)†	Average	Minimum	Maximum
Hourly rate	11	$56	$24	$125
Annual salary	25	$92,931	$6,000	$250,000
Production	33	34%	7%	80%
Collection	25	36%	12%	100%

*Data from American Dental Association Survey Center.[24]

†Percentages do not equal 100 because the compensation arrangements of some respondents did not fit into any of the four categories.

agement responsibility with no capital investment or financial risk. The disadvantage for the associate is little control over certain practice parameters and potential conflicts with the owner over patient and practice philosophy as well as constraints on professional judgment. Additionally, the associate in a sole proprietorship practice usually receives little or no liability, medical, disability, or life insurance or retirement benefits. On average, an associate may expect to earn $92,000 annually as an employee or an independent contractor.[24] Compensation for new associate dentists is negotiable and is paid based on an hourly wage, salary, percentage of production, percentage of collection, or incentives (usually a guaranteed minimum compensation with incentive increases for productivity) (Table 1-4).

Destination: Saudi Arabia

David Okuji, DDS, MBA

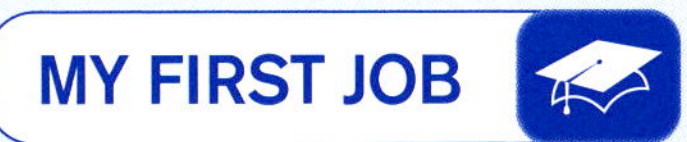

Life's twists and turns can surprise you and take you in directions you never would have imagined. In dental school, I assumed that I would graduate, pass the state board exam, and start a long career in private practice. I naïvely imagined settling into private practice, getting married, buying a house and a great car (not necessarily in that order), starting a family, and joining the local Rotary club. Little did I know that life's events would change my path toward happiness.

I did graduate, pass the board exam, get married, settle into a private practice, and buy a house. I was practicing as an independent contractor dentist, and my plan was to associate for a few years, then buy the practice from the owner. During the first 4 years of practice, I honed my clinical skills, improving my efficiency and the quality of my work. I developed my chairside manner so I could advise patients with a voice that exuded professional knowledge and confidence. In short, I learned the business of dental practice.

By the fifth year I knew that I did not want to buy the practice I was in, but I had no idea what to do next. I had invested 4 years in that practice without earning any equity. One option was to find another associate position, but I worried that would just be more of the same. Another option was to buy or start a new practice, but I would have to borrow a large sum of money, which seemed pretty risky.

During this period of uncertainty, I read an article in my dental society's newsletter about a new member who had just returned from a 5-year posting in Saudi Arabia. It was an intriguing story. I called the dentist to learn more about his experience in Saudi Arabia, and he warmly invited me to meet for lunch. My new colleague was friendly, outgoing, and hospitable. He described the relaxed work environment, the lifestyle in a foreign country, the excitement of world travel, and *the tax-free income.* That's right, the Internal Revenue Service provided income tax exclusion for United States citizens who worked abroad, and the government of Saudi Arabia didn't have an income tax. And, even more incredibly, the Saudi Arabian company was actively recruiting more US-trained dentists.

After a long discussion with my wife, we decided that this was a career opportunity worth investigating. I contacted the company, submitted my application, and read every book I could find on Saudi Arabia. Three months passed before my application went into final review, after which they finally invited me to join the company. I needed a week to deliberate before I could accept or decline the offer. It was definitely one of the longest weeks of my life. Not much sleep. Lots of stomach acid. Plenty of prayer. The week passed, and we made the decision to accept the position.

We spent 5 years in Saudi Arabia, and our daughter was born there. We forged many lifelong friendships, the work environment was relaxed, and the Saudi Arabian lifestyle was quite enjoyable. We traveled around the world multiple times in various directions. Our daughter saw every corner of the world as a child, and all the income I earned was almost entirely tax-free.

Upon returning to the US, I was fortunate to find a private practice to purchase in my seaside community. I loved it and practiced there for the next 20 years. The only thing I didn't do was to join the Rotary club.

In hindsight, I clearly see that my dental school dream of the perfect career path came true. It just took a 5-year detour through Saudi Arabia. The take-home lesson to my story is that there is no hurry to settle down and buy a practice. I was 10 years out of dental school before I bought a practice, and I still had a happy 20-year career in private practice.

As an associate, be sure that the employment contract clearly indicates whether your status is an employee or an independent contractor because there are significant tax implications.

Employee versus independent contractor status

As an associate dentist, determining whether you are a wage-earning employee or an independent contractor is financially critical because it directly impacts net income and income taxes. As an employee, the owner is responsible to withhold certain federal and state amounts from wages and to contribute certain federal and state taxes on the employee's behalf. Alternatively, an independent contractor is considered self-employed and therefore is paid the full amount of compensation and is personally responsible for estimating and paying all federal and state amounts due. It is strongly advised that an employment contract clearly indicate whether the associate's status is an employee or an independent contractor. The Internal Revenue Service (IRS) has rules and guidelines that define the independent contractor arrangement, and it may closely scrutinize the employment arrangement. Professional advice is required to draft the independent contractor agreement because the financial repercussions of a successful IRS challenge to the arrangement can be heavy. Even a contract researched and written by legal and accounting professionals can be successfully challenged and disallowed by the IRS. Box 1-2 provides some useful guidelines for potential indicators of employee or independent contractor status.

Owner dentist

Purchasing a practice

Purchasing a practice is a package deal: You get the good and the bad of the existing practice. There is immediate opportunity for generating revenue, but making any significant changes takes time and money.

Compared with starting a practice from scratch, purchasing a practice has the advantage that an existing patient base is purchased along with the practice, and there is a good likelihood that revenue will be generated immediately. However, the disadvantage is that nearly all of the seller's

Box 1-2 Guidelines for determining employee or independent contractor status

Potential indicators of employee status

The hiring dentist:

- Furnishes supplies, instruments, equipment, and/or office support
- Repairs instruments and equipment
- Formulates care guidelines and specifications
- Imposes safety precautions
- Determines and requires adherence to practice patient care management and methods
- Observes patient treatment methods
- Interprets patient care plans and treatment
- Can alter patient care plans and treatment
- Prohibits associate dentist from working for others, and/or associate dentist provides services on substantially full-time basis
- Assumes liability stemming from employee performance (through insurance or otherwise)

Potential indicators for independent contractor status

The hiring dentist:

- Lacks control over manner of performance
- Lacks authority to supervise the performance of a dentist contractor's work
- Lacks authority to terminate contract unilaterally without cause

The associate dentist:

- Controls premises or shares with hiring party
- Is compensated without reference to time engaged
- Provides and pays for all insurance including liability, unemployment, and workers' compensation
- Has the authority to delegate work to another dentist
- Has ownership of practice
- Possesses special professional skills
- Furnishes own instruments and equipment or leases them from hiring party
- Controls his or her employees
- Pays or shares employees' compensation
- Is obligated to reimburse hiring dentist for losses or damages

creation is purchased as well, which includes office design, choice of equipment, and selection of employees. If any of these are not to your liking, it takes time, money, and effort to change them. The existing employees' expectations and attitudes may never be changed. You also have to assume a great level of financial risk, manage all aspects of the practice, accept the maximum personal responsibility, incur a large amount of initial debt, and be available for patient emergency coverage 24 hours a day.[25] See chapter 3 for more information about purchasing a practice.

Texas Hold 'Em

Scott Stafford, DDS, MBA

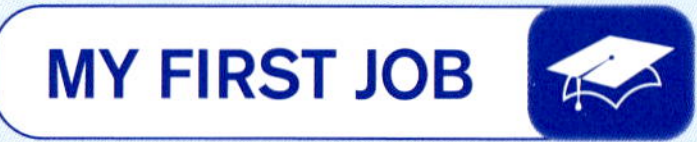

During my third year of dental school in Texas, I became acquainted with a local dentist who had a very prominent practice in town. I shadowed him throughout the year and observed him and his associate, who was only a couple of years my senior. Toward the end of that year, the owner offered me an associateship upon my graduation, which included the opportunity to purchase one-third of the practice after 1 year of associating. I had always wanted to own my own practice or a portion of a practice. This appeared to be the perfect opportunity to learn from a successful local dentist as well as fulfill my desire of equity in a practice. We signed the contract, and I felt miles ahead of my classmates.

During my fourth year in school, I continued to visit the office and gain as much information about my future position as possible. I also often visited with the associate dentist, and I tried to extract as much of his insight as possible. He was offered the same deal for employment and eventual partial ownership as I had been. He and I had long discussions about the purchase options.

After graduation, I began my associateship as agreed upon in our contract. I gained valuable experience in patient care and clinical efficiency during my time there. We had an in-house laboratory, which helped me hone my laboratory communication skills.

After approximately 6 months, the owner and I started discussions regarding the buy-in. The price was set at one-third of the annual gross income. For this I would receive one-third of the practice. There was no negotiating on the terms. For what I would be paying, I felt that I could start my own practice with 100% ownership. There was considerable growth in our area, and I decided to build my own practice rather than pay for the right to work with someone else. I finished out the remaining 6 months of my contract and used the time to study every aspect of a thriving practice. I learned everything from how to submit insurance claims to how to treat–or not to treat–staff. The associateship was invaluable, but I chose to start up my own practice because I wanted full ownership and the ability to set the course of my practice.

New practice startup

Starting a new practice as the sole proprietor is another way to enter private practice. Many new graduates rule this option out because such a venture is high risk, and they already carry a large amount of educational debt. But, starting from scratch has its advantages. For example, you have a high level of control over all aspects of the practice, including office design, equipment, and selection of employees. In short, the practice fits your vision. A startup practice, however, may experience an initially slow rate of cash flow because the patient base must be built from the ground up. See chapter 4 for more information about starting a new practice.

When you start up a new practice from scratch, you can make the practice fit your vision. However, you must be financially capable of withstanding an initially slow rate of cash flow because the patient base must be built from the ground up.

Conclusion

There are many positions to be played in the game of dentistry. The aim of this chapter was to familiarize you with the options available and help you analyze your motivation, abilities, and skills to help you determine which is best for you. The most important thing, however, is to get on the playing field. As the authors' stories showed, the first position you take may not be the one you keep throughout your career, but it will offer you valuable experience and insight that will eventually lead you to where you need to be.

References

1. Laise E. Odds-on imperfection: Monte Carlo simulation financial-planning tool fails to gauge extreme events. Wall Street Journal. May 2, 2009. http://online.wsj.com/article/SB124121875397178921.html. Accessed 28 December 2009.
2. Census bureau projects U.S. population of 305.5 million on New Year's Day [news release]. Washington, DC: US Department of Commerce; December 29, 2008. http://www.census.gov/Press-Release/www/releases/archives/population/013127.html. Accessed 29 December 2009.
3. Dow Jones Industrial Average. Yahoo! Finance website. http://finance.yahoo.com. Accessed 15 March 2009.
4. United States Department of Labor, Bureau of Labor Statistics website. http://data.bls.gov/cgi-bin/surveymost. Accessed 15 March 2009.
5. Bank of America. Practice sales & purchases. http://www.bankofamerica.com/vehicle_and_personal_loans/index.cfm?template=practice_sales_and_purchases. Accessed 12 August 2009.
6. Matsco. Practice acquisition & start-up financing. http://www.matsco.com/dentists/practice-financing-programs/practice-start-up-financing.htm. Accessed 12 August 2009.
7. Henry Schein Dental. Practice start-up. http://www.henryschein.com/us-en/dental/services/Financial/PracticeStartup.aspx. Accessed 12 August 2009.
8. GE Healthcare Financial Services. Practice acquisition finance. http://www.gehealthcarefinance.com/OurSolutions/LandingPages/GE_Practiceacquisition.aspx. Accessed 12 August 2009.
9. Gregory S. Dentists: Smiling in the face of recession. TIME. http://www.time.com/time/business/article/0,8599,1879760,00.html. Accessed 12 August 2009.

10. American Dental Association Survey Center. Distribution of Dentists in the United States: Historical Report, 1993 to 2001. Chicago: American Dental Association, 2003:1,14,15,60.
11. Defense Finance and Accounting Service. 2009 Military Pay Tables. http://www.dfas.mil/militarypay/militarypaytables/2009MilitaryPayTables.pdf. Accessed 30 September 2009.
12. US Public Health Service. The USPHS Dental Corps. Dental Recruitment Newsletter: Opportunities for New Graduates [2007-7.doc]. 2007;1(1):2. Available at: http://www.phs-dental.org/depac/newsletters/. Accessed 30 September 2009.
13. Van Pelt L, US Public Health Service. Indian Health Service dental program: Imagine your ideal career. Dental Recruitment Newsletter: Opportunities for New Graduates [2007-7.doc]. 2007;1(1):4. Available at: http://www.phs-dental.org/depac/newsletters/. Accessed 30 September 2009.
14. US Department of Health and Human Services, Health Resources and Services Administration website. Answers: NHSC LRP service requirements. http://answers.hrsa.gov. Accessed 29 December 2009.
15. Health Resources and Services Administration, National Health Service Corps website. Facts & figures. http://nhsc.hrsa.gov/about/facts.htm. Accessed 29 December 2009.
16. Paratus S, US Public Health Service. United States Coast Guard dental program. Dental Recruitment Newsletter: Opportunities for New Graduates [2007-7.doc]. 2007;1(1):6. Available at: http://www.phs-dental.org/depac/newsletters/. Accessed 30 September 2009.
17. Hickey D, US Public Health Service. Bureau of Prisons dental program. Dental Recruitment Newsletter: Opportunities for New Graduates [2007-7.doc]. 2007;1(1):5. Available at: http://www.phs-dental.org/depac/newsletters/. Accessed 30 September 2009.
18. University of North Carolina School of Dentistry website. Academic Dentistry. http://www.dent.unc.edu/careers/career_options/academicdent.htm. Accessed 5 October 2009.
19. Haden NK, Weaver RG, Valachovic RW. Meeting the demand for future dental school faculty: Trends, challenges, and responses. J Dent Educ 2002;66:1102–1113.
20. American Dental Association Council on Dental Practice. Associateships: A guide for owners and prospective associates. Chicago: American Dental Association, 2005:4.
21. American Dental Association Survey Center. 2004 Survey of Dental Practice–Income from the Private Practice of Dentistry. Chicago: American Dental Association, 2004:2–3.
22. American Dental Association Survey Center. Distribution of Dentists in the United States by Region and State, 2003. Chicago: American Dental Association, 2005:52.
23. Halley MC, Lalumandier JA, Walker JD, Houston JH. A regional survey of dentists' preferences for hiring a dental associate. J Am Dent Assoc 2008;139:973–979.
24. American Dental Association Survey Center. 2002 Survey of New Dentist Financial Issues. Chicago: American Dental Association, 2003.
25. American Dental Association Council on Dental Practice. Starting Your Dental Practice: A Complete Guide. Chicago: American Dental Association, 2007:18.

Finding a Job

Michael Okuji, DDS, MPH, MBA

David Okuji, DDS, MBA

This chapter is about finding your first job. It explores the job market, how to find a job, and how to land a job. Lastly, it presents issues that should be addressed upon taking a job as an associate dentist. The chapter is also about social skills and how to connect with others–important factors in finding your first job. School is a youthful, insular environment that is focused on education and technical skill. Life outside of academe is *never* student focused. Employers don't unconditionally love you like a parent or professor. You have to convince them that you are the best fit for their needs and then perform your best to meet them.

Life outside of school can be a shock to new graduates, who must learn different ways to connect, communicate, and work with others.

This chapter applies most directly to those who are choosing to start their career working for someone else; the next two chapters address purchasing a practice and starting a new practice, respectively. However, there is general advice regarding how to present yourself to the world and interact with others that is universally helpful to individuals starting out in the "real" world.

The Job Search

You know that after graduation you need to find a job. However, there are no signs to guide the way to finding that first job out of dental school. In the past, the first job was most often with the family dentist, where the setting was comfortable and familiar. But today, it is more common for new dentists to find employment within a multisite group practice, where team interaction is a fundamental part of the environment. To find a job in this setting requires a different set of technical and social skills.

Getting Started

The best time to begin looking for a job is during your junior year of dental school.

When you begin your search, start early because finding a job is a job in and of itself. The junior year of dental school is the best time to begin looking. Approach the search in earnest. Serendipity and perseverance certainly play a major role in finding a job, but luck is always with those who are prepared. Prepare, rehearse, and be ready to respond.

To get started, get some business cards and personal stationery printed, and don't skimp on paper costs. High-quality paper looks more professional than inexpensive, multipurpose paper. On both the cards and the stationery, list a local mailing address and an easily accessed telephone number, such as a cell phone number. Don't make a potential employer engage in phone tag.

Next, prepare your resume. Preferably keep it to one page, and definitely do not make it longer than two pages. It isn't an autobiography. Provide your contact information at the top of the page, followed by your education information, including postgraduate training, continuing education courses, and study clubs. Next, list any previous employment that is directly relevant to the job. Finally, list any volunteer activities and awards. Keep it clean, concise, and easy to read.

Every resume you submit should be accompanied by a cover letter tailored to that specific position.

For each job to which you are applying, prepare a cover letter on your personal stationery to accompany your resume. Never submit a resume without a cover letter, and never use a boilerplate (ie, standardized) cover letter. Tailor each cover letter to the job at hand. Make it personal, sincere, and, above all, professional. Avoid slang, shorthand email-type language, and contractions. If you aren't a very good speller, have a professor or grammatically inclined friend, family member, or classmate review your resume and cover letters before you send them out.

Finally, obtain a letter of recommendation that you can include with your resume and cover letter. Ideally, the letter should have specific reference to you being clinically proficient, teachable, and a reliable team player. Lacking that, seek a letter of recommendation that speaks highly of your work habits and personal ethics.

You never know when you could be talking to someone who could be your connection to a position, so don't be shy—tell everyone you meet that you are looking for a job.

Above all else, get the word out that you are looking for a job. Tell everyone you meet. Don't be shy. Liberally hand out business cards, because you never know when and where you'll make that connection that gets you a job. Continually widen your circle of influence, and be prepared to immediately follow up with a telephone call, resume, and cover letter and to be available for an interview.

Personal Referral Resources

Dental school professors

Professors are the first and best resource in a job hunt because they are usually near and easily accessible. Cultivate them while still in school. Most of the clinical faculty are in private practice and have a wide circle of friends in private practice. Most are also members of the local dental society, and some may even routinely employ graduates as associates in their office. Part-time, volunteer floor instructors are the best bet.

Professors are the first and best resource in a job hunt because they are usually easily accessible and naturally inclined to help their students.

Approaching current or former instructors doesn't have to be intimidating. They are there to help you succeed. Ask them to join you for a cup of coffee, and start by inquiring about how they found their first job and how they would start a job search in today's market. Ask for their perspective on topics such as opportunities in their neighborhood and employment in corporate practices.

After each conversation, be sure to let your instructor know that you appreciate his or her time, experience, and wisdom, then follow up with a letter of thanks. Once you graduate, make sure you give these instructors a business card, then follow up with a courtesy call in the months following.

The family dentist

Go out of your way to make contact with your family dentist while you're still in school. Family dentists are excellent resources because they know you personally and may introduce you to their circle of professional colleagues. Family dentists are usually willing and even flattered to talk to a dental student or new graduate about dentistry and jobs. Make a short courtesy call or visit and leave a business card. Be exceptionally courteous to the receptionist, because she controls the portal to entry and often exercises influence over office matters. Don't expect to meet with your dentist at this point; instead, arrange a meeting at your dentist's convenience, then follow up with a courtesy call or letter. At the meeting, find out how your dentist found his or her first job, and ask how you should approach a job search today. If the family dentist routinely hires associates, ask what characteristics he or she seeks, but don't ask for a job; just follow up with a letter of thanks.

Family dentists are excellent resources because they know you personally and may introduce you to their circle of professional colleagues.

Friends, family, and dental school colleagues

Don't underestimate the importance of keeping in contact with your dental school peers. Sometimes the only way to get a prized position is to know the right people.

Friends, family, and dental school colleagues can widen your circle of influence and should be kept apprised of your job search. Distribute business cards among them so they can easily pass them along to others. It is especially important to keep in touch with dental school peers, who may share tips, rumors, and referrals. If you attend a dental society meeting or continuing education course, make it a point to sit next to someone you don't know. Let him or her know you are a new graduate seeking employment and hand out a business card. Don't be shy. Your social and professional networks are a good bet in the job search because dental jobs, including most sole proprietor associate positions, are sometimes only softly marketed through word of mouth. Most prized jobs are never advertised.

Fire sale

fire sale
When a dentist or his or her family must sell a practice immediately due to ill health, disability, or death.

On occasion there is a dental practice fire sale, which occurs when a dentist or his or her family must sell a practice immediately due to ill health, disability, or death. These practices quickly lose value every day they are closed because patients find other dentists. Fire sales are broadcast by word-of-mouth, and news spreads quickly within the tight circle of community dentists. Expanding the circle of people who know you're looking for a practice and having your financial records prepared in advance (as described in chapter 1) make it more probable that you'll be the first to know and quickly close a sale on a fire sale practice.

Having your financial records prepared in advance can be a key advantage in trying to close quickly on a fire sale.

Public Resources

Classified advertisements

If you're having trouble finding a job through a personal referral, turn to the classifieds. Dental school alumni associations list open job positions on their school websites. The American Dental Association, California Dental Association, and other state associations regularly publish available job listings. Multisite group practices like Aspen Dental prominently advertise in the *Journal of the American Dental Association*. For positions that sound interesting, perform an analysis of the listing company through the Internet to learn how these multisite group practices present themselves to the public. Send a cover letter and resume to those that seem to be a fit.

Government agencies

Government agencies often have dental programs that hire new graduates. For example, the San Francisco Department of Public Health hires dentists for its Child Health and Disability Prevention Program, and it also staffs the dental section of the Jail Medical Service and geriatric division of Laguna Honda Hospital. These San Francisco venues are traditional starting positions for new dental graduates in California, and public health dentistry (as described in chapter 1) provides a great starting point for new dentists in any geographic region. You will find that the Internet is an excellent resource in the search for government employment.

Corporate group dental practice

Corporate dental practice has a presence throughout the United States, with every large city and metropolitan center having a multisite group dental practice. Western Dental Centers and West Coast Dental are multisite group dental practice employers in Southern California, and Pacific Dental Service and Bright Now Dental Network are management service organizations that employ dentists for affiliate group practices. You can find a group practice through journal advertisements or an Internet search, but be forewarned that these practices aren't for everyone. Expect to find a high-volume practice that prizes production.

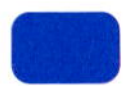

The Interview

Interviewing for a job requires a set of social skills significantly different from those used in dental school. Effective communication and interaction are much more important than intellect in the wider world, and to be persuasive without arrogance is an art that requires practice.

Nonverbal Cues

Eye contact with a confident demeanor is fundamental in an interview.

Nonverbal cues include posture, appearance, and hygiene. Wearing the appropriate clothes for the occasion is the first nonverbal cue. Each region has its own flavor. A suit is appropriate in one region but pretentious in another. Nevertheless, neatness counts in all cases. The shoeshine, haircut, and manicure send a positive nonverbal message, while denim, décolletage, sweats, sandals, and strong cologne or perfume send a negative message and are never appropriate. Eye contact with a confident

Important Questions to Ask at a Job Interview

Compensation

- ❑ Will I be an employee or independent contractor?
- ❑ Will I receive a salary, percent of production, percent of collection, incentive, or a combination of these types of compensations?
- ❑ Are prophylaxis and radiographs included in the production figure?
- ❑ Is personal protective wear provided?
- ❑ Are paid holidays, paid vacation, paid sick time, 401k, medical insurance, and liability insurance provided?

Office management

- ❑ Whom will I report to?
- ❑ Is a dental assistant assigned?
- ❑ Who will take the radiographs?

Patient base

- ❑ Does your practice accept patients with health maintenance organizations (HMOs), preferred provider organizations (PPOs), Medicaid, or Medicare?
- ❑ What are the number and mix of patients on any given day?
- ❑ Does your practice treat adults as well as children?

Duty and responsibility

- ❑ Will I be responsible for the examination, diagnosis, treatment plan, and case presentation of patients?
- ❑ Must I follow a treatment plan created by another dentist?
- ❑ Who does the periodontal charts, and who is responsible for signing and submitting them?
- ❑ Who does the prophylaxis, scaling, root planing, and curettage?
- ❑ What type of restorative, operative, fixed, and removable procedures are performed at your practice?
- ❑ Are extractions, root canals, and periodontal surgery performed as well?
- ❑ Is nitrous oxide, oral sedation, or intravenous sedation used?
- ❑ Who administers oral and intravenous sedation?
- ❑ Who prescribes medication?

Hours of operation

- ❑ What are the minimum and maximum working schedules available per day and week?
- ❑ Are there required evening and/or weekend hours?
- ❑ What is the emergency coverage requirement?

Insurance billing

- ❑ Are procedures billed under the treating dentist or the office name?
- ❑ If I am the treating dentist, who signs the claim?
- ❑ Who reviews billing procedures?

Contract

- ❑ May I see a sample contract?
- ❑ What are the employment terms and termination policies?
- ❑ Does "hold harmless" apply?

Fig 2-1 Checklist of questions to ask at a job interview.

demeanor is fundamental in an interview. Also, be sure to shake the interviewer's hand when leaving the interview.

Verbal Cues

Verbal cues start with the liberal use of politeness–courtesy is never out of style. Listen so that you will understand, and be especially solicitous to the receptionist. The hierarchy of an office is not always attributed to title, and the locus of decision-making power is sometimes hard to determine. Many times it resides in the staff rather than the dentist. Moreover, the manner in which you engage those around you speaks volumes about yourself. You are there to do a job, so leave your hubris at the door. Practice with mock interviews so you can present your case with conviction and ease during the real deal. You should also know the strengths and weaknesses of your resume by heart and address each to satisfy the needs of the potential employer.

While on an interview, be kind and courteous to all you encounter in the office—the staff is often influential in hiring decisions.

Answering and Asking Questions

Be prepared to answer questions about how you can contribute to the needs of the practice. How does your experience and skill fit the mission of the office? How can you give your lack of experience and proficiency a positive spin? Flexibility in time and work habits is often a key attribute that new dentists can offer a practice.

In return, be prepared to ask hard questions about the position. This interview is your opportunity to fully understand the job being offered. Prepare a list of questions about the job before you present for the interview. Some areas to explore are the hours, duties, responsibilities, and compensation (for ideas, see the checklist in Fig 2-1). You don't want any surprises the first day on the job.

Remember that the interview is as much your chance to find out about the position as it is the employer's chance to find out about you.

Starting a Job As an Associate Dentist

In a new job there are issues that a newly hired dentist should immediately address. There are the basics, such as befriending the office staff members by showing them courtesy and respect rather than treating them as your inferiors. Then there are the sticky details that present themselves as you try to determine the subtle differences between your role as an associate dentist and that of the owner dentist.

As an associate dentist, it is essential, but often difficult, to understand where the employer's responsibilities end and yours begin.

The owner dentist provides the dental setting, staff, and patients. He or she sets the hours, terms, and scope of service. In some settings, the owner dentist also sets treatment plan guidelines and may examine the patient and develop the treatment plan. Meanwhile, the associate dentist is a licensed professional responsible for clinical decisions and entrusted with the welfare of his or her patient. So, the question is, "Where is the line drawn between an employee taking direction and a licensed professional using clinical judgment?" Some important issues for an associate dentist to consider, especially in multisite group practices, include:

- Are you professionally responsible for clinical chart maintenance and appropriate and acceptable care?
- Are procedures that are billed to an insurance company substantiated by chart entries and supported by the patient's record?
- What area of control is the exclusive prerogative of the employer?
- What area of control is the exclusive prerogative of the treating dentist?
- In some settings multiple dentists treat the same patient. In these circumstances, is there a signed treatment plan and consent?
- Under the same circumstances as the previous question, will treatment quality be uniform among the dentists in the office?
- Are you professionally responsible for a safe practice environment, including sterilization protocol, personal protective equipment, and radiation exposure?
- Are the instruments clean and sterile?
- Are the assistants employing universal precautions?
- Is proper radiation safety being practiced?
- What controls are there for proper billing procedures under the signature of the treating dentist?

Although associate dentists are at-will employees, they are also licensed professionals who are ultimately responsible for treatment decisions and outcome. Every year the California State Dental Board responds to a handful of complaints regarding substandard or inappropriate care provided by associate dentists. A recent case involved the revocation of the dental license of an associate dentist in a multisite group practice for gross negligence and incompetence based on inadequate record keeping, insurance fraud, failure to diagnose or treat, and excessive treatment. In this particular case, the dentist testified that the employer set the tone for aggressive treatment, eg, placing 30 fillings in one appointment. In an older California case the associate dentist treated a child who was sedated with an untoward outcome. The dentist had inadequate training in sedation management and worked in the absence of the anesthetist. In both cases the associate dentists were the treating dentists and therefore at risk, even though they testified that they were working under the standard protocol of the office. Both cases ended in license revocation. Although the Board investigates only a few egregious cases each year, there may be many more unreported cases.

The bottom line remains that the associate dentist must refuse to engage in actions he or she deems unwise and unsafe for the patient, even at the risk of termination of employment. Some questions to ask about a patient's treatment plan include:

- Is the health history complete?
- Do radiographs, charting, and other records support the treatment plan?
- Do you agree with the treatment plan, including:
  - Type of procedure
  - Number of total procedures
  - Number of procedures in a single appointment
  - Length of the appointments
  - Selected anesthetic

If you don't feel comfortable with the practices of your employer, confront the situation or leave the practice, but do not jeopardize your license and the health of your patient. You, not the owner dentist, will be held responsible in any resulting malpractice suits.

If you are uncomfortable with any aspect of the chart and/or treatment plan, you must confer or decline to proceed. You, as the treating dentist, are responsible for providing appropriate and safe treatment within your capability. The ethical issues of beneficence and nonmalfeasance always apply. Any untoward treatment outcome is the responsibility of the treating dentist, not the managing dentist or the owner. The employee-employer divide ends at the dental chair.

Following are additional considerations that apply specifically to small private practices and corporate dentistry.

Small Private Practice

As an associate dentist in a small private practice, be prepared to treatment plan like the employer, remembering that patients will be comfortable with the style of the office and owner dentist. A newly found diagnosis after a period of stability or an elaborate treatment plan may seem to be a reflection of your inexperience. The aggressive new dentist stands

In a small private practice, remember that patients most likely have a personal relationship with the owner dentist, so it is important to emulate his or her style until you build trust and familiarity with the patients.

Table 2-1 Corporate dental entities that employ or support dentists*

Company	Annual revenue (US $, in millions)	Number of locations
American Dental Partners	350	–
Birner-Perfect Teeth	65	–
Bright Now	350	225
Interdent	250	185
Pacific Dental Services	190	110
Heartland Dental Care	160	174
Western Dental Centers	150	115
Affordable Dental Care	150	120
Dental Care Alliance	120	77
Dental One Partners	110	67
Aspen Dental	90	88
Great Expressions Dental Centers	70	65

–, unavailable.
*Data from Raffel.[1]

to lose patient trust, so watch and learn from the owner. However, if you feel patients are being mistreated, the same directive as above applies: confront the dentist or leave the practice.

Corporate Dentistry

A large corporate-owned dental practice is characterized by a centralized management company that provides organizational and administrative support for multiple dental office locations over a large geographic area. The myriad permutations of the legal, business, practice, and licensing aspects of these dental entities are dizzying and beyond the scope of this text. In simple terms, these corporate-owned practices can be organized as a health maintenance organization (HMO) or a dental management service organization that provides financing and support but is not licensed to practice dentistry. Table 2-1 lists some of these large corporate dental entities that employ or support dentists. For illustration, the following case example gives a real-life view of one multisite group dental practice, Western Dental Centers, based in Orange, California.

Case example: Western Dental Centers

Western is a multisite HMO with offices in California, Arizona, and Nevada that employs a large number of dentists. Western provides dental services to its own HMO enrollees and no other HMO. Western contracts with most PPOs and accepts patients on Medicaid in California's DentiCal program. It is also a Healthy Family Plan (California) provider, accepts all indemnity insurance, and offers an in-house credit plan. Western provides services to children, young adults, adults, and seniors as well as patients with disabling medical conditions or complex medical histories. Western also employs dentists who limit their practice to pediatric patients and have special expertise in treating patients with developmental challenges.

The associate dentist is the entry-level position for a new dentist. The associate reports directly to the managing dentist in the office, who then reports to the region's operations director, who is also a dentist. Within Western Dental Centers' structure, there is opportunity for promotion from associate doctor to managing doctor to regional operations director to vice president of operations.

Associates are employees of Western and are paid a daily wage for each day actually worked. Associates are not paid for holidays, vacation, or sick time. They are eligible for additional compensation beyond the daily wage based on a percentage of the production formula. Associates participate in Western's 401k program. Although Western provides liability insurance to its associates, medical insurance is not a benefit.

Associates execute a proprietary Western employment contract, with a minimum term of 1 year. Upon completion of the initial term, the con-

CORPORATE DENTAL ENTITIES

- American Dental Partners: www.amdpi.com
- Birner-Perfect Teeth: www.bdms-perfectteeth.com
- Bright Now: www.brightnow.com
- Interdent: www.interdent.com
- Pacific Dental Services: www.pacificdentalservices.com
- Heartland Dental Care: www.heartlanddentalcare.com
- Western Dental Centers: www.westerndental.com
- Affordable Dental Care: www.affordabledentalcare.com
- Dental Care Alliance: www.dentalcarealliance.net
- Dental One Partners: www.dentalonepartners.com
- Aspen Dental: www.aspendent.com
- Great Expressions Dental Centers: www.greatexpressions.com

tract is renewed automatically thereafter. After the initial term, the contract can be terminated at any time given a 30-day notice. Western reserves the right to terminate any associate at any time.

Western Dental Centers offices are open Monday through Thursday from 9 am to 8 pm, Friday from 9 am to 7 pm, and Saturday from 8 am to 4:30 pm. All offices are closed on Sunday. Associates typically work 5 days a week on an 8-hour shift that can start anywhere between 8 am to 11 am. Western allows some associates to work 6 days a week. Some associates also elect to work part-time from 1 to 4 days a week as they build their own private practice.

Associate doctors are assigned a dental assistant. Every office has a mix of dental assistants and registered dental assistants as well as a radiograph technician and a sterilization technician. Western does not employ dental hygienists or nurse anesthetists. Associates provide prophylaxis, scaling, curettage, and root-planing services.

On average, associates treat slightly more than 11 patients a day. In general, one-third of those patients are new and require an examination; one-third require "minor" treatment, such as fillings, crown delivery, and routine extraction; and one-third require "major" treatment, such as root canal treatment and crown preparation.

All dentists in the office perform examinations and case presentations. Associates perform nonsurgical and surgical extractions and nonsurgical root canal treatment on all teeth, including molars. Each associate determines when a procedure is within his or her capability and is subject to the restrictions imposed by the managing dentist or Western's Quality Management department.

Most Western offices have a general dentist who limits his or her practice to extraction and an oral surgeon and periodontist who only provide specialty surgery. Some Western patients are referred to out-of-office specialists. Nitrous oxide is available in almost all Western offices, and associates are expected to administer nitrous oxide when appropriate. Oral sedation and intravenous sedation are not available in Western's offices.

Conclusion

Like an athlete who stays with one team until retirement, some dentists will make a career out of the first position they take. Most dentists, however, will change jobs at least once, and many will change as often as professional athletes are traded from team to team. Either way, your first position will set the tone for your career and influence the eventual path of your career, so plan thoroughly and plan early.

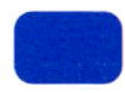

Acknowledgment

Thank you to Louis J. Amendola, DDS, Chief Dental Director and Vice President of Recruitment at Western Dental Centers, who provided the information about the operation of Western Dental Centers.

Reference

1. Raffel E. Truths not myths about a DMSO. American Association of Dental Consultants. http://aadc.org/site/pdf/dmso-truths.pdf. Accessed 20 July 2009.

Purchasing a Practice

David Okuji, DDS, MBA
Francis Serio, DMD, MS, MBA

This chapter takes the reader through the key steps of buying an existing dental practice. It addresses how practices are bought and sold, evaluating a practice for purchase, determining a fair practice price, and understanding purchase documentation.

As discussed in chapter 1, the primary reason to buy a functioning practice is the immediate cash flow this option provides. This can be a critical factor if your personal financial situation includes a school loan and/or a home mortgage payment. A practice purchase also provides an established telephone number and location and access to an immediate source of patients, although some patients may leave during the transition of ownership. Another reason to buy a practice is that it saves you the time and trouble associated with starting a practice from scratch, allowing you to focus on practicing clinical dentistry right away. However, this advantage may be short lived if the protocols in place are not to your liking and you end up having to work around them or change them.

The key thing to remember is that when you purchase a practice, it is a package deal that includes tangible assets such as staff, equipment, and the facility, as well as intangible assets such as reputation and philosophy. At the beginning of the purchase process, it is important to thoroughly study the practice philosophy and standards of patient care to ensure that they are compatible with your vision. Radical changes to the way the practice is run may upset the staff and drive patients away. If possible, it is best to keep the existing staff when purchasing a practice because patients often identify more with the staff than with the dentist, but remember that it's also possible to inherit low-performing staff. Taking over

When you purchase a practice, you are purchasing everything that goes along with it—the location, patients, staff, equipment, facility, reputation, and philosophy—so make sure you can live and work with what you're getting.

the existing facility and equipment can also be a mixed blessing, depending on their state of repair, vintage, and quality. In short, if you have decided that purchasing a practice is the best option for you, it is extremely important to do your homework to make sure that the one you buy is the one you want.

How Practices Are Bought and Sold

Brokered Sales

Dental journals and dental school websites have classified sections that list dental practices for sale through a dental practice broker. The dental practice broker listed in the journal represents the seller and prepares, advertises, and markets the practice. The broker works like a real estate broker, ie, meets the potential buyer, distributes practice information, leads the property inspection, negotiates the sale terms, and prepares the sales agreement. Some offer financing through preferred lenders. The broker may require the potential buyer to execute a confidentiality or nondisclosure agreement before releasing practice documents and may also prohibit a buyer from contacting the staff until a certain point in the negotiation is reached. This allows the owner to continue normal operations and assures that the staff and patients don't become prematurely concerned about their future with a new owner.

The practice broker may also act as the seller's appraiser, ie, determine the price of the practice. As with a real estate transaction, the practice price is based not only on the tangible assets but also on a host of other intangible factors such as the location, the quality of the patient base, and the professional reputation of the doctor, which will be discussed in more detail later in this chapter and in chapter 7.

When purchasing a practice, it is wise to retain your own representation rather than relying on the seller's broker.

The real estate analogy is apt. A practice broker is required to have a state real estate license or to be an attorney. The broker's fee is received from the seller as a percentage of the sale, and, as in a real estate transaction, the broker may represent both the buyer and the seller. However, it is in the buyer's best interest to retain separate representation. The buyer's representative should participate in all the aspects of due diligence (described later in this chapter) and the negotiation. The buyer's representative has an integral role in evaluating the purchase agreement and can initiate a practice search as well as inquire about a purchase opportunity. The representative can also contact a dentist who is nearing retirement and is ready to transition to retirement but has not put thought into action. This is often an overlooked source of practices for sale.

Private Sales

The owner can place his or her practice for sale without a broker, a method that is also used in real estate. An owner can advertise a private sale in the same journals and dental school websites as a broker, and, often, the staff members aren't informed of the impending sale. An owner-represented practice sale often initially lacks the proper documentation and preparation required for full disclosure to the buyer, but, nevertheless, the seller must be prepared to deliver all the relevant documents in a timely manner and provide unfettered access to the office and records for inspection. It's important to note that owner-represented sales can be slower and more contentious because of the lack of an intermediary representative.

Buying a practice through a private sale by the owner can be more difficult and time consuming than going through a broker.

Fire Sale

An exception to a routine sale of a dental practice is a fire sale, also discussed in chapter 2, which is the immediate sale of a practice due to an unanticipated situation. It may be that the seller is unable to carry on the practice and recognizes that practice value quickly dissipates each day that it is closed, or, in many cases, the unexpected death of a dentist may drive a fire sale. This type of sale is spread by word of mouth among the dental community. If your strategy is to buy a practice by fire sale, be prepared to act immediately and have all of your financial information and documents ready at hand.

Evaluating a Practice

There must be a balance between the value of immediate cash flow and the work needed to bring the practice up to your expectations in order for a practice purchase to make sense. There is no such thing as the perfect practice, but the buyer must not be overeager to purchase a practice that will later breed dissatisfaction or buyer's remorse.

Ask yourself whether the location is right for you and whether the asking price seems right. Do you know why the practice is for sale? Will it fit your needs in terms of office size? What is the practice's yearly revenue?

You can always expect the seller to put a higher value on a practice than a buyer, but also be prepared to walk away from the deal if the numbers don't make sense.

The length of time the practice has been on the market can be a good indicator of its value. Practices that are outdated, overpriced, poorly equipped, ill maintained, or disadvantageously located or that have low revenue or poor financial records are slow to sell. Junk is junk even at a "good" price, unless there is an obvious potential upside that makes the purchase worthwhile—especially at a discount.

Due Diligence

due diligence
Research and analysis performed in preparation for a business transaction.

If you find you're still interested in purchasing a practice after an initial evaluation, begin an in-depth analysis. A recent graduate is encouraged to seek experienced counsel at this stage. In a practice purchase the buyer is entitled to see all of the practice's financial records, clinical performance records, and physical facility. When purchasing a practice, it is important to review these records and perform your due diligence. Due diligence means that a buyer makes a focused effort to verify the seller's representations of all aspects of the practice, whether it be the lease, production, expense, staff, charts, or quality of care. Anything that impacts the practice, patient retention, and expected future revenue is subject to due diligence. Don't be shy. It's not being rude or nosy. It's business, not personal, and it's important.

Performing your due diligence means that you're prepared to ask hard questions. The best way to start is to prepare a detailed checklist, then call the seller's broker. Request supporting documents and expect expedient delivery of those documents, as well as answers to your questions and a resolution of all of your concerns. The list of financial information needed for a thorough analysis is formidable (Fig 3-1), but it is important to be thorough.

It is also always prudent to perform your clinical due diligence (Fig 3-2). Review patient charts to assess the quality of recorded examination information, radiographs, treatment plans, treatment notes, financial notes, consent, completed Health Insurance Portability and Accountability Act (HIPAA) release forms, and other documentation. Examine a few patients at random if possible; it may be enlightening.

Finally, investigate the physical facility (Fig 3-3). Remember, buyer beware! The buyer owns the visible, unseen, and unforeseeable problems in the practice once the deal is done.

Financial Due Diligence Checklist

- ❑ 3 to 5 years of federal tax returns. (Tax return forms vary depending on whether the practice is a sole proprietorship [Schedule C]; partnership, limited liability corporation, or C corporation [Form 1120]; or subchapter S corporation [Form 1120S]. Most dental practices are a sole proprietorship and file a Schedule C.)
- ❑ 5 years of financial statements, including a year-to-date income statement, balance sheet, and statements of cash flow.
- ❑ Production by provider and types of procedures.
- ❑ Aged accounts receivable.
- ❑ Fee schedule and a 5-year summary of fee increases.
- ❑ A fee report for the local area (if available).
- ❑ Managed care insurance adjustments to revenue.
- ❑ Annual expenses by category and as a percentage of revenue. (This total can be found on the income statement if it is properly categorized; the higher the overhead percentage, the lower the relative value of the practice.)
- ❑ Laboratory expenses for 5 years and year-to-date, as well as the history of remakes.
- ❑ Office hours and number of days open per week and weeks per year.
- ❑ Associate dentist agreements, if any.
- ❑ Employee list and dates of hire and compensation, including fringe benefits, work hours, and responsibilities.
- ❑ Manuals: office, Health Insurance Portability and Accountability Act (HIPAA), and Occupational Safety and Health Administration (OSHA).
- ❑ Third-party managed care contracts and fee schedule.
- ❑ Total revenue itemized to cash, insurance, managed care contract, and Medicaid.
- ❑ Seller's practice valuation, methodology, and the credentials of the valuation preparer.

Fig 3-1 Checklist of financial information needed for a thorough analysis of a dental practice for sale.

Clinical Due Diligence Checklist

- ❑ Total number of active patients seen in the past 12 to 18 months.
- ❑ Number of new patients per month for 5 years and year-to-date. (Beware of the seller who has lost momentum in the practice and allowed the practice to languish. Annual revenue should be steady or increasing.)
- ❑ Number of patients with insurance and their insurance plan types (ie, indemnity, PPO, capitation, and other managed care plans).
- ❑ Patient demographics, especially age, sex, and family income.
- ❑ Number of appointments, efficiency, and revenue for the hygiene department. The hygiene team should produce about three times its cost.
- ❑ Accurate breakdown of the type and number of treatment procedures performed.
- ❑ Accurate breakdown of procedures referred out of office.

Fig 3-2 Checklist of clinical information needed for a thorough analysis of a dental practice for sale.

Physical Facility Due Diligence Checklist

- ❑ Office blueprints.
- ❑ Evaluation of the floor plan.
- ❑ Video, photographic, or virtual images of the facility. (Has the practice had a recent facelift or are the furnishings and fixtures tired and outdated?)
- ❑ Copy of the lease.
- ❑ Duration of the lease.
- ❑ Lease renewal amendments.
- ❑ Lease assignment. (Can it be assigned to a new tenant or must it be renegotiated?)
- ❑ Inventory of the office equipment.
- ❑ Inventory of the dental equipment, including dates of purchase, depreciation, and maintenance records.
- ❑ List of physical items currently in the facility but not included in the sale.

Fig 3-3 Checklist of information about the physical facility needed for a thorough analysis of a dental practice for sale.

What Is Being Purchased?

The purchase price should be for the practice as it currently exists and not for any potential developments. Every practice has both tangible and intangible assets.

Tangible assets

Tangible assets in a practice purchase include the dental and office equipment. The initial cost, depreciation, and maintenance log should be available. These items are subject to appraisal to assign a fair market value with the general assumption that equipment retains approximately 25% of its value after depreciation, assuming it is in good shape. Dental and office supplies on hand are included if they have not expired. The lease and renewal amendment is a critical, tangible asset to the purchaser and financial lender, and the value of leasehold improvements may be included in the purchase price.

Accounts receivable

accounts receivable (AR) The money for services owed to the practice but not yet collected.

Accounts receivable (AR) is the money for services owed to the practice but not yet collected. Some AR can be outstanding insurance payments or patient payment plans. AR age, so note how long they've been outstanding, their turnover, and/or how long it has taken to collect them. Although AR are tangible assets, they are often excluded in the practice purchase. If AR are included in the purchase price, a current aged AR report is necessary; any accounts in arrears should be purchased at a substantial discount or disallowed altogether. An account more than 120 days past due is considered uncollectible. Also, if a practice has a significant old AR balance that has slow turnover, it is wise to analyze its business system to determine why these unpaid balances exist. You should also find out who is responsible for refunds on previous claims and overpayments.

Accounts receivable are often excluded from the purchase price; however, if they are included, any accounts in arrears should be substantially discounted or disallowed because it is questionable if they will ever be recovered.

Intangible assets

Intangible assets include goodwill and future cash flow. One definition of goodwill is the difference between the appraised value of the hard assets and the selling price, which is usually the value placed on future revenue. The seller almost always has a higher expected value for goodwill than the buyer. Future cash flow depends as much on the buyer's effort as on the current financial condition of the practice; therefore, future cash flow is generally based on the retention of the current cash flow.

goodwill
The difference between the appraised value of the hard assets and the selling price, which is usually the value placed on future revenue.

Practice Valuation

The price that property would sell for in the open market is called fair market value.[1] It is the price that is agreed upon between a willing buyer and a willing seller. Neither party is required to act, but both parties must be reasonably aware of all relevant facts.[1]

fair market value
The price that property would sell for in the open market between a willing buyer and a willing seller.

Determining the fair market value of a dental practice is as much an art as a science. It is imperfect at best. Because there are many different ways to value a practice, it is incumbent upon the buyer to become familiar with the seller's valuation methodology and be prepared to obtain an independent valuation. Valuation methodology ranges from the relatively simple and straightforward to complex calculations. All valuations are subjective to a degree, depending on assumptions such as the value of equipment, fixtures, and furnishings (ie, tangible assets) and the expected rate of growth and value of goodwill (ie, intangible assets). See chapter 7 for more information about performing a practice valuation of both intangible and tangible assets.

Find out what valuation methodology the seller is using to obtain the asking practice price, and be prepared to obtain an independent valuation.

Interestingly, the value of a practice may depend in part on the psychologic makeup of the buyer. A prospective buyer who has the temperament and personality to start a practice from scratch will see less value in buying an existing practice than a second buyer who has less business confidence. The seller's practice is then more valuable to the second buyer, which is a decided advantage for the seller.

There is no regulation of valuation analysts, although there are professional appraisal organizations. The National Association of Certified Valuation Analysts, Institute of Business Appraisers, and the American Society of Appraisers provide training, continuing education, and certification of valuation professionals. To find a valuation analyst or appraiser certified by one of these organizations, visit their websites.

Projecting Revenue and Operating Income

net revenue
Actual money collected minus refunds.

operating expense
An expense that is directly associated with producing income.

operating income
Revenue minus operating expenses.

EBITDA
Earnings before interest, taxes, depreciation, and amortization (ie, operating income).

The key to all of these valuation methods is the projection of the revenue and operating income to the buyer. Net revenue is the actual money collected minus refunds, and operating income is revenue minus operating expenses. An operating expense is an expense that is directly associated with producing dental income. Interest on practice loans, business taxes, depreciation of practice equipment, and the amortization of intangible assets are not operating expenses. In finance, operating income is called EBITDA (earnings before interest, taxes, depreciation, and amortization). Usually the federal income tax Form 1040 for a sole proprietorship Schedule C is analyzed to determine the net operating income by adding back nonoperating expenses, which are taken as deductions on the tax return. These nonoperating expenses are discretionary by the seller and are "added back" to gross revenue for the prospective buyer's use. Some of these addbacks include:

- Discretionary expenses for the direct benefit of the owner (like compensation to officers)
- Depreciation
- Interest
- Charitable contributions
- Pension and profit-sharing plans
- Commissions
- Conferences and conventions

PROFESSIONAL APPRAISAL ORGANIZATIONS

- National Association of Certified Valuation Analysts: www.nacva.com
- Institute of Business Appraisers: www.go-iba.org
- American Society of Appraisers: www.appraisers.org

- Dues and subscriptions
- Medical insurance
- Medical expenses
- Meals and entertainment
- Pension administration

Cross-checking the income tax return entries with the office bank statement entries is an excellent check and balance for an accurate picture of the office net operating income. See chapter 7 for further details.

Acceptable Value of a Practice

There are a number of ways to determine the value of a practice. Common methods for evaluating and determining ranges of acceptable prices are the market sales approach, capitalized earnings approach, and investment yield approach.[2] See Appendix I for sample valuations of two practices using these approaches.

Market sales approach

The market sales approach utilizes historical sales of similar dental practices to determine the value of a practice. Dental practices are traditionally priced from 50% to 100% of their annual net revenue. This approach bundles tangible and intangible assets. The trend line of the intangible assets must be considered because the value decreases if factors such as location, practice reputation, and patient flow are decreasing over time. The market approach gives you a broad view of the seller's asking price compared with the price of most dental practices. It is based on historical sales and doesn't take into consideration the dynamics of the current market. The market sales approach places the asking price on the high end of the market.

The market sales approach is based on historical sales figures and generally places the asking price of the practice on the high end of the market.

Capitalized earnings approach

The capitalized earnings approach determines value in relation to financial risk and reward. This approach also bundles tangible and intangible assets and is based on the following equation:

The capitalized earnings approach determines value in relation to financial risk and reward.

$$\text{Fair market value} = \frac{\text{Operating income} - \text{Dentist compensation}}{\text{Capitalization rate}}$$

Box 3-1 Example of an estimated capitalization rate

Average stock market return at valuation date	20.51%	
Risk premium for size of business	+ 3.00%	(Return required by buyer)
Risk specific to practice	+ 5.00%	(Based on practice parameters)
Expected long-term practice growth rate	– 3.00 %	(Based on annual fee increase)
Capitalization rate	25.51%	

Capitalization rate

dentist compensation A reasonable wage that would be paid to another dentist to provide the dental service for the practice.

capitalization rate Sum of the average market return at valuation date, risk premium for size, and the risk specific to the practice, minus the estimated long-term growth rate of the practice revenue.

Dentist compensation is a reasonable wage paid to another dentist to provide the dental service for the practice, but determining a capitalization rate is more complex. It comprises the sum of the average market return at valuation date, risk premium for size (ie, the additional return required to attract an investor to a small company), and the risk specific to the practice, minus the estimated long-term growth rate of the practice revenue (Box 3-1).

The risk specific to the practice is influenced by many factors, a majority of which are subjective:

- Gross income
- Location
- AR
- Lease terms
- Retention of staff
- Competition
- Transferability
- Patient type
- Profitability
- Growth potential
- New patient volume
- Equipment
- Repeat visits
- Size of patient base
- Service mix

Therefore, the calculation of the capitalization rate has an inherent degree of subjectivity.

Investment yield approach

The investment yield approach demonstrates the ability of the practice to potentially pay a dividend to the buyer.

The investment yield approach demonstrates the ability of the practice to potentially pay a dividend to the buyer. The investment yield is determined by calculating the return on investment (ROI):

$$\text{ROI} = \frac{\text{Operating income} - \text{Clinician compensation}}{\text{Initial investment}}$$

The initial investment is the practice purchase price. A table can demonstrate the investment yield (ROI) based on a range of purchase prices. Depending on the buyer's risk tolerance, a spreadsheet can run a comparison of ROI between different practices or within a single practice to determine what purchase price point meets the investment ROI objective.

The market sales, capitalized earnings, and investment yield approaches may also be used in tandem to bracket the acceptable range of the purchase price of a specific practice (see Appendix I).

Other Dental Practice Valuation Methods

A multitude of other dental practice valuation methods can also be employed.

Income approach

The income approach (also called the *present value approach*) using the discounted cash flow (DCF) formula is a good valuation method because it calculates the present value of expected future earnings from an existing practice. Both the current and expected future cash flows are essential reasons to buy an existing practice. The calculation is a bit sophisticated because it is based on a DCF, which calculates the time value of future earnings over a specific time period, then discounts the money back to today's present value. It requires assumptions on the expected cash flow and the capitalization rate, which is discussed in more detail in chapter 7.

The income, or present value, approach calculates the present value of expected future earnings from an existing practice.

The present value is easily determined using expected net earnings estimates and an appropriate discount value. The difficulty is estimating the proper number for each factor in the equation. The income approach estimates the value of the intangible asset of goodwill, then adds the fair market value of the practice's tangible assets, such as equipment, to determine the total fair market practice price.

Estimators

Variations of the market sales approach are the multiple of the gross revenue estimator and the multiple of earnings estimator. Because of their ease of use, these estimators–based on historical sales of similar practices–are commonly used to evaluate the value of dental practices. However, the gross revenue estimator is not very useful because it is net income that the buyer is purchasing, not the gross revenue. High gross revenue with a high overhead expense means that the buyer is working hard for little return.

The multiple of earnings estimator is a more reliable valuation method than the gross revenue estimator because it is based on net operating income, rather than gross revenue, and it considers the past 5 years rather than only the year immediately prior to sale of the practice.

Multiple of earnings, also called *multiple of net operating income*, is a more meaningful metric. A 5-year average operating income is used instead of the previous year's performance because a seller may ramp up production in the year prior to a sale to try to increase the value of the practice. The range of multipliers of either gross revenue or earnings is based on the current condition of the practice and the current state of the economic environment.

The caveat with any percent estimator is whether the estimator accurately reflects the return the buyer will receive. In other words, can a percent estimator, which is a static figure based on the historical performance of similar practices in the area, accurately predict the future performance of the practice in a fluid and changing environment and economy?

The Sale Contract

A good dental sale contract clearly describes what is being purchased, the responsibility and expectation of each party, and the time frame in which the expectations are to be executed.

Once the buyer and the seller agree on the purchase price, a practice sale contract is drafted and reviewed by both parties' attorneys. A good dental sale contract–like a good real estate contract–clearly describes what is being purchased, the responsibility and expectation of each party, and the time frame in which the expectations are to be executed. A dental practice broker can provide a draft from a boilerplate practice sale contract. The buyer and the seller review and modify the draft so that the terms of the contract meet mutual needs. It is strongly recommended that both the buyer's and seller's attorneys review and revise the contract to protect each individual's interests.

General topic headings used in a practice sale contract include:

- Parties involved and the date of the contract
- Time and place of sale
- Total purchase price
- Allocation of purchase price in consultation with an accountant
- Goodwill value and allocation in consultation with an accountant
- Payment of purchase price
- Security for purchase
- Phase-out agreement

- Noncompete clause
- Risk of loss
- Duty to maintain supplies
- Custodian of records
- Transfer of records
- Use of seller's name
- Prorate insurance, utilities, taxes, and laboratory expense
- AR management
- Tax ramifications in consultation with an accountant
- Rework, re-treatment, and refund of fees for previous dental treatment
- Hold-harmless agreement
- Seller's warranties and representations
- Buyer's warranties
- Life and other insurance
- Warranty on equipment
- Contingencies
- Appointment of escrow agent
- Prorated costs and expenses like wages
- Entire agreement
- Binding on heirs

Other documents that are usually part of the sale contract include:

- Bill of sale: Transfer of the title of the property sold to the buyer
- Existing lease assignment: Assignment of the office lease to the buyer
- Release: Release of the seller from office lease liability
- Promissory note: Written promise by buyer to pay any amount borrowed in a seller-financed purchase
- Security agreement: Security of the promissory note with collateral of the assets transferred against the claim of other creditors
- Employment or independent contract agreement: Contractual agreement if the seller is hired back after the sale
- Real estate property sales contract: Separate contract if the dental office facility is also purchased

References

1. Internal Revenue Service. Determining the Value of Donated Property. Washington, DC: United States Department of the Treasury. Publication no. 561. Published April 2007. http://www.irs.gov/publications/p561/ar02.html#d0e139. Accessed 27 July 2009.
2. Hill RK. Transitions: Navigating Sales, Associateships & Parternships in Your Dental Practice. Chicago: American Dental Association, 2006.

Starting a New Practice

Francis Serio, DMD, MS, MBA
David Okuji, DDS, MBA

Many dental students start school knowing they want: *(1)* to provide dental care and *(2)* to "be their own boss." Although these words flow easily from the lips of students, most have little–if any–experience in the business world. Starting a practice moves the practitioner from the realm of health care professional to that of entrepreneur and small business owner with all of the attendant challenges and rewards. For example, practitioners must realize they are selling two things, time and service, and time is the more valuable commodity. Time cannot be replaced. That which is not accomplished now will be accomplished later with a corresponding debit of time. Therefore, one of the most important aspects of running a successful dental practice is efficient scheduling and management of the dentist's time.

Starting a practice from the ground up is both rewarding and challenging. The primary reason to start a practice from scratch is to have total control over the design and function of the practice. Detailed planning and realistic expectations are the key factors to success in a startup. Comprehensive research and planning takes time, so it's important to plan while you're still in school or during residency, even though finishing the educational program is still uppermost on your mind.

Detailed planning and realistic expectations are the key factors to success in a startup practice.

Getting Started

First and foremost, the hardest part of establishing your own practice is just getting off the starting blocks. But as in any race, it's good to get a head start, so if you are planning to start a practice from scratch, here are some items to get you off and running:

1. Write down your goals; having them in mind is not the same as committing them to paper.
2. Formulate a plan of action around these written goals. Remember that to enter into business means that you must be organized, able to earn a profit, and willing to live a lifestyle that will sustain a practice that meets the needs of patients as well as the financial obligations to staff, suppliers, lenders, and yourself.

The Break-Even Point

business break-even point
The point at which a business begins to make a profit.

family break-even point
The point at which a family has enough income to meet its needs.

The next step toward getting in business is determining what your break-even point is. The business break-even point is the point where a business begins to make a profit. It's equally critical to calculate the family break-even point, which takes into consideration how much income the practice needs to allow the family to reach its goals. Some break-even factors to consider are:

- Family size
- Type, size, and cost of the family home
- Type and cost of automobiles
- Educational costs, whether public or private school (including college)
- Entertainment costs (eg, vacations)
- Charitable contributions or church support
- General living expenses
- Retirement planning
- Resources for other investments

Establishing a Location

Choosing a good location is key for the success of the practice as well as the happiness of the family.

The first three axioms of real estate purchase are location, location, location, and they are the same axioms to consider when starting a practice. Location is in part a family decision based on the proximity to relatives, lifestyle choices, schools, economic factors, and other personal wishes. These family goals translate to business decisions as well, so as you explore geographic areas, you'll need to consider their potential as locations for a successful practice. Once you've established a general location, determine the demographics of the area and the distribution of local dentists. Start by talking to the local chambers of commerce, banks, and local or state dental associations. Dentist and population ratios and the trends of both for more than 5 years may give some indication of the potential growth for a new practitioner in the community. New home and school starts, existing home sales, and industry or business startups in the area may also give an indication of the vitality and relative youth of a community. See chapter 1 for more insight into geographic goals and objectives as part of your career strategy.

Building a Business Plan

There are some things common to dental practice, whether you are starting from scratch or buying an established practice. Chief among them is the need to acquire the backing to fund the purchase or buildup of a practice. Paramount to acquiring funding is the development of a well-conceived business plan. The old adage "Failing to plan is planning to fail" is appropriate here. Many practitioners point to their comprehensive business plans as the reason they were able to obtain financing on favorable terms and achieve success during their first year as neophyte business owners. In addition to a practice business plan, it also may be necessary to prepare a personal balance sheet and a 5-year projection of *pro forma* cash flow (see chapter 7).

Many practitioners point to their comprehensive business plans as the reason they were able to obtain financing on favorable terms and achieve success during their first year as new business owners.

Buying Versus Renting Office Space

One major decision in starting up a practice is whether to rent or buy the office space. The advantage to rental space is that there is no long-term commitment: It is easy to move if the practice outgrows the current space, and there is increased cash flow because rent is less expensive on a monthly basis than a mortgage on a building. The disadvantage of rented space, however, is that there is no equity built, and you may have to cover the costs of leasehold improvements that will ultimately become the property of the landlord. There could be rent increases, which may be larger than expected, and the lease may not be renewed.

Advantages of renting: No long-term commitment is required and cash flow is increased.

Disadvantages of renting: No equity is built, value of any improvements is not retained, and unexpected rent increase or lease termination is possible.

The advantage to purchasing office space–or an entire building for that matter–is that equity appreciation is realized. Of course, this assumes there is a strong real estate market. It's also easier to modify the space, al-

Advantages of buying: Equity is built, modification of space is easier, renting or selling property is possible if the practice moves, and cost of the property may be shared with another professional tenant.

Disadvantages of buying: Space may be too small and initial and ongoing costs may be high.

though it could be difficult to add space depending on the building and configuration of the surrounding area. It's also possible that the property could be rented or sold if the practice moves, and there is the potential to share the cost of the property with another professional tenant. The disadvantage to purchasing office space or an entire building could be that the space is potentially too small, that the initial cost is high, and the ongoing costs could be higher than a comparable rental space.

Once you've made the lease/buy decision, you'll need to make further decisions regarding the design of the office space and the purchase of equipment for the practice. Large dental supply companies often have office design resources, and there are some builders who work in conjunction with dentists and provide advice and expertise in starting a practice. In any case, be sure that the builder you've chosen has experience in dental practice construction. The build-out process of installing operatory utilities, nitrous oxide plumbing, and other features unique to dental practice goes more smoothly with a seasoned hand.

Equipping a Practice

Don't fall into the trap of buying too much too soon. Just get the necessities and add on as patient volume and revenue increase.

One danger associated with starting a practice is ending up with unsustainable fixed costs. This is usually caused by equipping too many operatories at the outset or buying all of the expensive, high-technology armamentarium available to clinical dentistry. When you start fresh, certain items, such as an electronic dental record-keeping system, financial control package, electronic insurance filing system, and digital radiology equipment, are necessities. But other high-ticket, high-technology items can wait until you've established a profit.

Operatories are equipped as patient volume and revenue increase; to initially equip operatories that are underused means that the equipment may rapidly depreciate without any revenue generation. Do not succumb to the heavy-handed sales pitch of your friendly dental sales representative. Financial performance and service mix dictate when certain items should be purchased. Assume that whatever plan you choose, the final cost will be 15% to 20% higher than what you initially budgeted.

Resources for Starting a Practice

Starting a new practice requires the support of many outside resources. First, identify the resources that will help you build your office:

- An interior design firm or dental supply company for office space planning and design
- A real estate professional to help with leasing or buying office space leasing
- A dental supply company for dental equipment and supplies
- Banks or lending institutions for financing

Next, identify the resources that will help you operate the office:

- Personnel agencies, advertising, and word of mouth for staff recruitment
- Dental practice consultants for business consultation
- Accounting and legal counsel
- Companies performing equipment maintenance and repair

Once the practice is up and running, it may be worthwhile to hire an office manager to assume the day-to-day challenges of running the business. It does not mean that the principal owner in the practice does not know everything about the business side of the practice; rather, it means that someone else takes care of the myriad office details, which leaves you available for precious treatment time.

Once the practice is up and running, it may be worthwhile to hire an office manager to assume the day-to-day challenges of running the business, although it is important to remain aware—and ultimately in charge—of how your business is run.

Startup Business Costs

Attracting patients to the new practice and consequent cash flow may be a slow process depending on the practice location and unmet demand for dental care in the community. Plan to finance not only capital expenses but also operational expenses out of pocket for several months.

Box 4-1 presents sample assumptions and demonstrates how to estimate the cost of starting up a dental practice.

Box 4-1 Sample cost estimate for a startup dental practice

Sample assumptions:

- Dental office size: 1,200 sq ft for three operatories
- Gross lease rate: $2/sq ft ($2,400 monthly lease)
- Office design and project manager: $10,000
- Complete office build-out, including cabinetry and fixtures: $100/sq ft
- Equip and supply each operatory: $20,000
- Overrun: 10%
- Lender charges: 3% of the loan amount fees for 100% financing of the startup project

Calculations:

Design and project management	$10,000
Improvements and contractor's fee (1,200 sq ft × $100)	$120,000
Equipment and supplies (3 operatories × $20,000)	$60,000
Subtotal:	$190,000
10% cost overrun	$19,000
Subtotal:	$209,000
Working capital (based on a hypothetical pro forma cash flow)	$50,000
Financing required	$259,000
Lending fee (3% of total financing)	$7,770
Total cost:	$266,770

Avoiding Common Pitfalls

There are several ways that business owners often get themselves into trouble. Below are some tips for staying away from these pitfalls:

1. *Don't ignore business and management problems.* Some of these include:
   - Collection rates
   - Staff interactions
   - Condition of the facility
   - Employee accountability
   - Expense control
   - Nonpayment of bills or taxes

2. *Don't give up total control to the office manager.* An office manager can be useful because he or she will afford you more time to focus on providing high-quality dental care. However, never cede complete business control to a single individual because more than one office manager has found a way to dip into practice money when the owner was not paying attention.
3. *Be sensitive to patient needs and desires.* Depending on the location of the office and patient expectations, it may be necessary to expand your available services by taking continuing education courses. Not having the necessary skills to provide sophisticated services such as esthetic dentistry procedures sends patients elsewhere. In addition, provide convenient office hours and make sure your office is accessible.
4. *Have a clear idea of the market in which your practice operates.* It is sage advice for new practitioners to find an established mentor in the community; however, this may be more difficult in a small community where the new practitioner is viewed as competition.
5. *Plan for expansion.* As part of the business plan for the practice, the number of new patients should be estimated and–hopefully–realized going forward. As the practice gets busier, there should be a plan in place for service growth, an increased hygienist staff, and facility expansion. Many practices do not plan for an accompanying increase in availability of dental hygiene services for maintenance and treatment of mild to moderate periodontitis. This lack of planning to accommodate increasing patient volume is an indirect way of guaranteeing that the practice will never grow.

Conclusion

Starting a dental practice from scratch is a formidable task to be undertaken only by entrepreneurial and business-minded dentists. To design a practice that is located, designed, and run exactly to your vision is enticing, but it carries a high financial risk. You must design, furnish, equip, and staff the practice without a single patient waiting at the door, which places a premium on planning, budgeting, creativity, and diligence.

Insuring Your Practice and Yourself

Eric Studley, DDS

It is important to review your insurance benefits on a periodic basis to keep your plans up-to-date with your changing needs.

The importance of purchasing the correct insurance policies from knowledgeable insurance advisers became painfully clear to me following a dental career–ending personal disability, years of litigation against an insurance company and its agents, and astronomic legal expenses that had significant effects on my family and me. We place our patients on recall to monitor changes in their oral health, and we likewise should review our insurance benefits on a periodic basis to keep our plans current with our constantly changing lives.

This chapter introduces basic insurance coverage and terminology, including malpractice (professional liability), office and business, disability, health, and life insurances. It is important to choose plans in each area that will protect a rich income stream and the assets it produces. Equally important is choosing a good insurance adviser. As in dentistry, where there are specialists with a higher level of training and expertise in certain areas, there are insurance advisers who specialize in specific areas of insurance. Although one-stop shopping is convenient, you may be wise to seek counsel from separate advisers knowledgeable in each area of insurance.

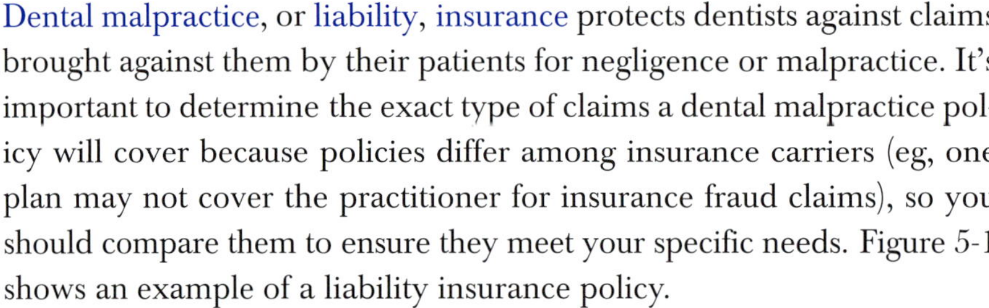

Malpractice (Liability) Insurance

dental malpractice (liability) insurance
Protects dentists against claims brought against them by their patients for negligence or malpractice.

Dental malpractice, or liability, insurance protects dentists against claims brought against them by their patients for negligence or malpractice. It's important to determine the exact type of claims a dental malpractice policy will cover because policies differ among insurance carriers (eg, one plan may not cover the practitioner for insurance fraud claims), so you should compare them to ensure they meet your specific needs. Figure 5-1 shows an example of a liability insurance policy.

A malpractice insurance carrier's financial rating is also important. This rating allows the consumer to measure the financial strength of the carrier, which affects the carrier's ability to pay claims and adjust premium rates. Rating services can be particularly useful for this purpose. Also note that a carrier endorsed by a dental association may offer a discount such as a lower premium if the insured passes a carrier-sponsored risk management course given online or through local societies.

Some carriers require a loss-run report on the insured, which gives information on past and current malpractice claims and litigation. It's quite simple to obtain malpractice insurance for the first time because there is no prior history of claims to investigate.

claims-made policy
Pays claims on the insured only when the policy is in force. This means that claims on service rendered while the policy was in force but filed after the policy was terminated are not covered.

A dentist has two options when choosing a malpractice policy: claims-made and occurrence. A claims-made policy pays claims on the insured only when the policy is in force (ie, you must continually keep your policy in force in case a claim arises from a previous or current year). A claims-made policy shouldn't be abruptly cancelled even if a dentist ceases to practice dentistry; instead, tail coverage (explained below) should be purchased at the time of practice cessation to cover the dentist for claims that could be filed after the dental practice closes.

occurrence policy
Pays claims on the insured for service rendered when the policy was in force, even if the claim is filed after coverage has ended.

Alternatively, an occurrence policy pays claims on the insured for services rendered when the policy was in force, even if the claim is filed after coverage has ended, so tail coverage is not required. An occurrence policy is initially more expensive than a claims-made policy, and not every

RATING SERVICES

- A.M. Best Company: www.ambest.com
- Standard & Poor's: www.standardandpoors.com
- Moody's Investors Service: www.moodys.com
- Fitch Ratings: www.fitchratings.com

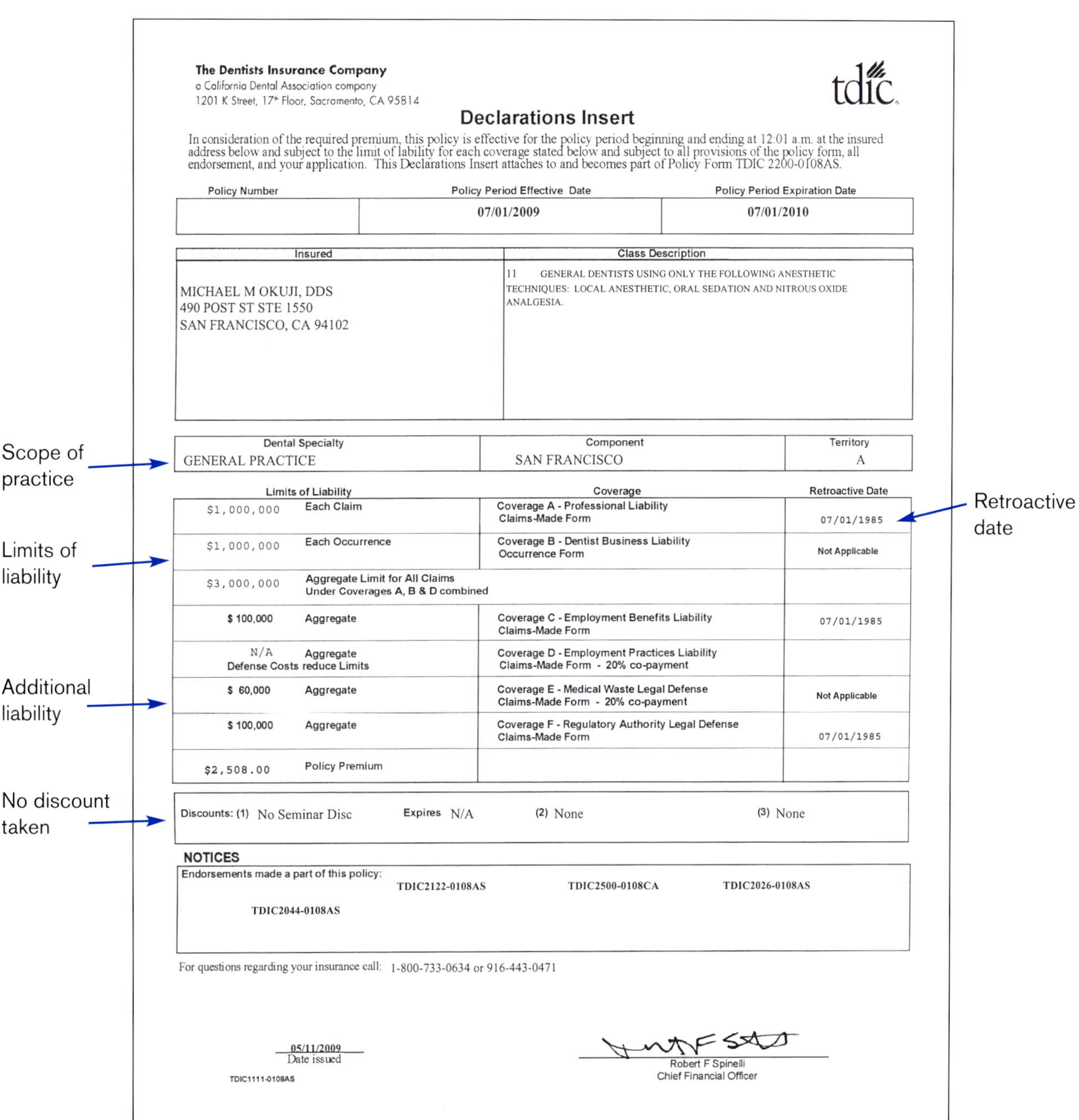

The Dentists Insurance Company
a California Dental Association company
1201 K Street, 17th Floor, Sacramento, CA 95814

tdic.

Declarations Insert

In consideration of the required premium, this policy is effective for the policy period beginning and ending at 12:01 a.m. at the insured address below and subject to the limit of liability for each coverage stated below and subject to all provisions of the policy form, all endorsement, and your application. This Declarations Insert attaches to and becomes part of Policy Form TDIC 2200-0108AS.

Policy Number	Policy Period Effective Date	Policy Period Expiration Date
	07/01/2009	07/01/2010

Insured	Class Description
MICHAEL M OKUJI, DDS 490 POST ST STE 1550 SAN FRANCISCO, CA 94102	11 GENERAL DENTISTS USING ONLY THE FOLLOWING ANESTHETIC TECHNIQUES: LOCAL ANESTHETIC, ORAL SEDATION AND NITROUS OXIDE ANALGESIA.

Dental Specialty	Component	Territory
GENERAL PRACTICE	SAN FRANCISCO	A

Limits of Liability		Coverage	Retroactive Date
$1,000,000	Each Claim	Coverage A - Professional Liability Claims-Made Form	07/01/1985
$1,000,000	Each Occurrence	Coverage B - Dentist Business Liability Occurrence Form	Not Applicable
$3,000,000	Aggregate Limit for All Claims Under Coverages A, B & D combined		
$ 100,000	Aggregate	Coverage C - Employment Benefits Liability Claims-Made Form	07/01/1985
N/A Defense Costs reduce Limits	Aggregate	Coverage D - Employment Practices Liability Claims-Made Form - 20% co-payment	
$ 60,000	Aggregate	Coverage E - Medical Waste Legal Defense Claims-Made Form - 20% co-payment	Not Applicable
$ 100,000	Aggregate	Coverage F - Regulatory Authority Legal Defense Claims-Made Form	07/01/1985
$2,508.00	Policy Premium		

Discounts: (1) No Seminar Disc Expires N/A (2) None (3) None

NOTICES

Endorsements made a part of this policy:
TDIC2122-0108AS TDIC2500-0108CA TDIC2026-0108AS
TDIC2044-0108AS

For questions regarding your insurance call: 1-800-733-0634 or 916-443-0471

05/11/2009
Date issued

Robert F Spinelli
Chief Financial Officer

TDIC1111-0108AS

Fig 5-1 Sample of a liability policy from the Dentists Insurance Company, a California Dental Association–affiliated company. The liability policy is written for a general dentist with a retroactive date of 7/1/1985. The limits of liability are $1 million for each occurrence and $3 million aggregate, and there is additional liability coverage for business, employment benefits, medical waste, and regulatory defense. A discount has been offered but not taken.

insurer will sell occurrence policies. These policies are hard to obtain and expensive to purchase, but some employer dentists may require that an employee dentist have an occurrence policy.

Other important terms to remember when purchasing a malpractice policy include limit of liability, tail coverage, retroactive coverage, renewal, settlement with and without a consent option, and territory.

Limit of Liability

limit of liability
The amount of malpractice coverage you have to protect yourself in the event that you are sued.

A limit of liability is the amount of malpractice coverage you have to protect yourself in the event that you are sued. Carriers offer limits of liability of $200,000/$600,000, $1 million/$3 million, or $2 million/$6 million. Currently, $1 million/$3 million coverage is the standard limit for a general practitioner, which means that the insured is covered up to $1 million per claim and $3 million aggregate per year. Liability limits are dictated by dental specialty, procedures performed, type of anesthetics utilized, employer requirements, and managed care contractual agreements.

Because one limit of liability is based on performed procedures, check with your state dental board to determine the definition of a "dental procedure." Most likely, procedures such as botulinum toxin type A (Botox) procedures are not included. In addition, because liability limits are dictated by employer requirements, and an employer pays for a claims-made policy, as an employed dentist you should determine whether your employer will continue to pay the policy premium or provide tail coverage if you terminate your employment.

Tail Coverage

tail coverage
Protects against any claim arising from past events after a claims-made policy is no longer in effect; usually purchased when a dentist retires or ceases to practice.

As explained above, the need for tail coverage is the principal difference between claims-made and occurrence policies. Tail coverage is usually purchased when a dentist retires or ceases to practice. This type of coverage protects against any claim arising from past events after the claims-made policy is no longer in effect. Some companies do not charge for tail coverage in the event you become disabled or if you've had continuous coverage for numerous years without a claim. Tail coverage may also be required when you switch malpractice insurance carriers, unless the new carrier offers retroactive coverage.

Retroactive Coverage

Retroactive coverage covers any claim that occurred while you were covered by your previous carrier, obviating tail coverage when changing claims-made policy malpractice carriers.

retroactive coverage
Protects against claims for services rendered while you were covered by a previous carrier, obviating tail coverage when changing claims-made policy malpractice carriers.

Renewal

Renewal of a malpractice policy doesn't automatically occur every year; instead, the carrier may send a renewal application that you must complete and return. It's important to pay the insurance premium (cost of the policy) on time because a late premium payment may adversely affect your policy renewal or trigger higher premiums. Changing your specialty also may cause nonrenewal.

renewal
Continuance of a malpractice policy from one period to the next. Renewal of malpractice insurance doesn't occur automatically, and events such as late payment of premiums or a change in specialty may cause nonrenewal.

Settlement with a Consent Option

A settlement with a consent option means that the insured retains the right to consent to settlement of any claim or suit. However, the carrier can't settle any claim or suit against you without your consent and is subject to an arbitration of the consent issue.

settlement with a consent option
The insured retains the right to consent to settlement of any claim or suit.

Settlement with No Consent Option

Settlement with no consent option means that the carrier has the right to settle or contest any claim or suit that is covered by your policy without your consent. If you agree to these terms, your carrier may reduce your policy premium.

settlement with no consent option
The carrier has the right to settle or contest any claim or suit that is covered by your policy without your consent.

Territory

Territory refers to the location where you practice, and it affects the cost of your policy premium. Cost varies by state, so do your research. Urban areas usually have higher premiums than rural locations. A new dentist who practices in different territories (counties) and states should seek a malpractice carrier that offers comprehensive coverage that includes all areas in which he or she practices.

territory
The location where you practice, which affects the cost of your policy premium.

Keeping Current

Keep your malpractice insurance policy current, which means notifying your malpractice insurance carrier when you change:

- Practice location
- Employers
- Tax filing status
- Ownership of a practice
- Number of staff, hygienists, and dentists, including specialists
- Performed procedures
- Types of anesthetics administered

Failing to do so could result in noncoverage of a malpractice claim.

Employed Dentists and Hygienists

An employee or independent contractor dentist who practices in an office may have to provide his or her own professional malpractice policy for that location.

An employee or independent contractor dentist who practices in an office may have to provide his or her own professional malpractice policy for that location. Usually the office will request a copy of the policy declaration page as proof of coverage. For hygienists, employees but not independent contractors are usually covered under the employer's malpractice policy. However, the premium for a hygienist malpractice policy is inexpensive and worth the cost for additional coverage.

What to Do When a Lawsuit Occurs

Lawsuits are served either personally or by certified letter with a mail-return receipt. If this happens:

- Accept the letter.
- Immediately notify your liability insurance carrier.
- Do not call the patient.
- Do not call the attorney representing the patient.
- Do not alter financial or clinical records.
- Do not talk to anyone except your attorney.
- Do not release any documents without discussing the claim with your attorney.
- Be truthful when discussing the case with your attorney.

Office Insurance

If you own your practice, it is imperative to protect the time and effort you've put into building that practice with the proper insurance. Inadequate coverage can cause irreparable financial hardship in a disaster. In addition, states mandate specific types of office insurance–consult with your attorney, accountant, or state government website to find out what coverage you are legally required to have. Also keep in mind that as your life changes, so will your professional and personal insurance needs; therefore, it is a good idea to consult with your insurance adviser throughout your career.

States mandate specific types of office insurance—consult with your attorney, accountant, or state government website to find out what coverage you are legally required to have.

Business Office Policy

Property and contents insurance

Property and contents insurance covers the loss of property and contents of your office if your office space is rented as well as the real estate if you own the property in the event of fire, theft, and other disasters. Disasters that are covered should be listed in the policy, but certain disasters, such as floods and earthquakes, may require separate coverage. It's important to acquire the most extensive coverage available in your area. Not all policies are the same, so review your options carefully before making a decision.

property and contents insurance
Covers the loss of property and contents of your office if your office space is rented as well as the real estate if you own the property in the event of fire, theft, and other disasters.

Umbrella insurance

Umbrella insurance is a situation in which one policy is enforced to cover more than one asset (eg, a home and automobile covered under one policy) and may result in a discount on the premium and eligibility for additional limits of liability in increments of $1 million. For example, if a car insurance policy has a $200,000 liability limit and a homeowner's policy has a $300,000 liability limit, a $1 million umbrella policy increases coverage to $1.2 and $1.3 million, respectively. It's also important to note that a business umbrella and a personal umbrella, which excludes all business assets, are separate policies.

umbrella insurance
One policy enforced to cover more than one asset (eg, a home and automobile covered under one policy); often associated with a discount on the premium and eligibility for additional limits of liability in increments of $1 million.

Business interruption insurance

Business interruption insurance pays for losses that occur and helps pay expenses if the business is unable to function because of a loss.

business interruption insurance
Pays for losses that occur and helps pay expenses if the business is unable to function because of a loss.

Employee-Related Insurance

Certain types of insurance are deemed mandatory by state law once you hire an employee. Consult your accountant, attorney, or state government website for specific details. You could receive state-levied fines and penalties for noncompliance.

Workers' compensation insurance

workers' compensation insurance
Mandatory employer-paid insurance that provides monetary and medical benefits to employees for any injury or illness that occurs as a result of the job, the most common of which in dentistry is a needle stick.

Workers' compensation insurance is a mandatory employer-paid insurance that provides monetary and medical benefits to employees for any injury or illness that occurs as a result of the job, the most common of which in dentistry is a needle stick. The benefits paid to employees can be short- or long-term, temporary or permanent; however, an employee may lose his or her right to receive benefits if a claim isn't filed within 2 years of the occurrence.

The state's workers' compensation board will determine the benefit amount an employee receives and can adjudicate a claim if a disagreement or dispute arises between the employer and insurance carrier. In that situation, the board has the final decision.

Your business entity can affect who is eligible for workers' compensation benefits, which means that sole proprietors, partnerships, independent contractors, and corporations all have different participation requirements. Verify which requirements apply to your practice with your accountant, attorney, or insurance adviser.

State disability insurance

state disability insurance
Provides coverage for employees who become disabled as a result of an injury or illness that isn't related to employment; required when the first employee is hired.

State disability insurance provides coverage for employees who become disabled as a result of an injury or illness that isn't related to employment, and it's required when the first employee is hired. Cash benefits are paid to replace lost wages, but these benefits don't cover medical expenses.

Employee dishonesty coverage (fidelity bond)

employee dishonesty coverage (fidelity bond)
Protects the employer from losses and damages to a business caused by the dishonest action of an employee.

Employee dishonesty coverage (fidelity bond) will protect the employer from losses and damages to a business caused by the dishonest action of an employee.

Employment practices liability coverage

employment practices liability coverage
Protects the employer from an employee's claim of wrongful termination, discrimination, and other employment-related claims.

Employment practices liability coverage protects the employer from an employee's claim of wrongful termination, discrimination, and other employment-related claims.

Disability Insurance

When you buy a car, you purchase automobile insurance, and when you buy a home, you purchase homeowner's insurance. These types of insurance cover major tangible assets in case of loss, so what about insuring yourself from a catastrophic disability, which could limit or prevent you from earning an income? You've invested considerable time and money to reach your professional goal, so now that you have finally reached that goal, it's important to insure your income stream.

There is a succession of disability insurance policies that you'll need throughout your career; some even argue that a disability policy is more critical than life insurance for a new practitioner. There are several factors that help determine the amount of coverage you need and qualify for, such as current income, expenses (including savings), expected future earnings, and other disability insurance in force, such as a group long-term disability plan.

There are several factors that help determine the amount of disability coverage you need and qualify for: current income, expenses (including savings), expected future earnings, and other disability insurance in force, such as a group long-term disability plan.

Underwriting and medical requirements apply to both life and disability insurance, which take current age as well as type and amount of coverage into consideration. A medical examination is usually required and involves a physical evaluation (sometimes administered by a paramedical examiner employed by the carrier at a location of your choice) as well as a complete medical history. You may be required to sign a consent form so the insurance carrier can access your medical history for the past 10 years through the Medical Information Bureau. The carrier may contact other health care professionals to obtain copies of your medical records to explain current or past conditions. They may also check your medication history. A pre-existing condition or ongoing medical problem doesn't necessarily hinder you from getting a new policy, but it may mean that you'll pay a higher premium. The carrier also may exclude certain medical conditions and reduce the benefit period, but not all carriers view conditions in the same way.

There are many factors to consider when designing the policy that is right for your particular situation, so it's important to understand all the options to make the correct choice, especially when weighing value, cost, and how you want the policy to perform.

Personal Disability Insurance

personal disability policy
Covers a loss of income in the case of limited, total, short-term, or permanent disability, which may be caused by an illness, injury, problem pregnancy, heart attack, depression, cancer, or diabetes.

A personal disability policy is one of the most important insurance policies to purchase. This type of insurance covers a loss of income in the case of limited, total, short-term, or permanent disability, which may be caused by an illness, injury, problem pregnancy, heart attack, depression, cancer, or diabetes.

Although this section lists and defines many of the parts of a disability policy, insurance terminology may vary across companies, and not all companies offer the same benefits and provisions mentioned below.

Issue and participation limits

issue and participation limits
The amount of disability benefits that can be purchased based on your profession and income.

Issue and participation limits relate to the amount of disability benefits that can be purchased based on your profession and income. Insurance companies do not share the same issue and participation limits, so it's critical to know and understand how the maximum benefits can be purchased.

Own-occupation disability policy

own-occupation disability
Pays benefits if you can't perform the material and substantial duties of your own occupation (ie, your regular occupation at the time of disability) because of illness or injury.

Own-occupation disability pays benefits if you can't perform the material and substantial duties of your own occupation because of illness or injury. *Your own occupation* refers to your regular occupation at the time of disability. You're considered totally disabled if you're unable to perform any work involved in your own occupation, even if you're able to perform unrelated work in a different occupation.

Benefit period

benefit period
The length of time a disability claim is paid.

The benefit period is the length of time a disability claim is paid (eg, 2, 5, or 10 years). Some carriers offer benefit periods that last until the policyholder reaches the age of 65 to 67 years as well as some form of lifetime benefit.

Noncancelable coverage

noncancelable coverage
Coverage that cannot be canceled as long as premiums are paid on time.

It is best to pursue policies with noncancelable coverage because disability coverage is pointless if it can be canceled when you need it most. To avoid this possibility, choose a policy that's noncancelable and guaranteed renewable to age 65 years as long as premiums are paid on time.

Guaranteed renewable disability policy

A guaranteed renewable disability policy is renewable for life as long as you pay your premiums and work full time. The best of these policies have no age limit for renewing. However, policy premiums may increase after age 65 years.

guaranteed renewable disability policy
Policy that is renewable for life as long as you pay your premiums and work full time.

Elimination period

An elimination period functions the same way a deductible does in other types of insurance. It is the period of time you must wait after becoming disabled before benefits begin, usually from 1, 2, 3, or 6 months to 1 or 2 years. Policies with long elimination periods have lower premiums for the same coverage.

elimination period
The period of time you must wait after becoming disabled before benefits begin.

Accumulation period

An accumulation period is a set amount of time in which enough days, weeks, months, or years of disability can accumulate to satisfy each elimination period. The accumulation period begins on the first day of disability. If you return to work after a period of disability that's shorter than your elimination period, but you become disabled again while you are still in the accumulation period, the time you were originally disabled still counts toward the fulfillment of your elimination period.

accumulation period
A set amount of time in which days, weeks, months, or years can accumulate to satisfy an elimination period.

Rider

A rider is an additional provision that is added to an insurance policy that adds enhanced features to the basic policy. Additional charges for a rider are added to the insurance premium.

rider
An additional provision with enhanced features that is added to an insurance policy.

Residual disability benefit rider

A residual disability benefit rider provides benefits for partial (ie, residual) disability. An illness or injury may not result in total disability, but it may limit your ability to work in your own occupation and may mean a decreased income. Or, you might have total disability and return to work but not at the predisability level of income. In either case, a residual disability benefit rider is critical.

residual disability benefit rider
Provides benefits for partial disability.

Future increase option rider

Obtaining additional disability coverage to protect a growing income normally requires proof that you're in good health. A future increase option rider allows you the option to purchase additional disability coverage each year up to the age of 55 years with no further medical insurability

future increase option rider
Allows you the option to purchase additional disability coverage each year up to the age of 55 years with no further medical insurability requirement.

requirement. This rider is a way to ensure that a growing income is protected regardless of a change in your health status, and your eligibility is determined by your current financial situation (ie, income and employment) and existing disability insurance protection.

Cost-of-living adjustment rider

cost-of-living adjustment (COLA) rider
Adjusts disability benefits to reflect inflation.

A cost-of-living adjustment (COLA) rider adjusts disability benefits to reflect inflation, which is often a forgotten economic factor when planning for the future. A COLA of 3% to 5% is usually offered at different premium levels.

Catastrophic disability benefit rider

catastrophic disability benefit rider
Offers added protection from the financial impact of a severe disability.

A catastrophic disability benefit rider offers added protection from the financial impact of a severe disability, such as one that results in cognitive impairment; the loss of two or more activities of daily living like bathing, continence, dressing, eating/feeding, toileting, and transferring; or irrecoverable loss of sight in both eyes, hearing in both ears, speech, or the entire use of both hands, both feet, or one hand and one foot. In combination with the basic disability policy benefit and any other disability coverage, the catastrophic disability benefit rider may pay up to, but not exceed, 100% of income from all sources.

Premium payments

Premium payments, including level and graded premium payments, are tailored by carriers to fit different financial situations. Some premium payment programs allow for additional discounts on a personal disability insurance policy, including multiple policy, preferred risk, an employer-sponsored plan, and nonsmoker discounts. These discounts vary by state and may not be offered by all carriers.

Level premium payment

level premium payment
Premium payment that remains the same up to the policy expiration date.

A level premium payment remains the same up to the policy expiration date.

Graded premium payments

graded premium payments
Premium payments that are lower at the beginning of the policy period and increase every year while the policy is in force up to age 50 years, at which time it is converted to a level payment.

Graded premium payments are lower at the beginning of the policy period and increase every year while the policy is in force, but they cost more over the life of a policy than a level premium payment. A graded premium payment is converted to a level premium payment as soon as it's financially feasible up to age 50 years. Upon conversion, the premium rate is set at the rate indicated for that age.

Important Questions to Ask When Choosing a Disability Insurance Policy

- ❑ How much is the monthly benefit?
- ❑ How soon after disability are benefits payable? (What is the elimination period?)
- ❑ How long should the benefit and the benefit period last?
- ❑ How do factors like current income and health influence the cost of my premium?
- ❑ Would a residual disability benefit rider be beneficial to me?
- ❑ How does the policy keep pace with inflation and expected future earnings?
- ❑ What is the difference between the future increase option and cost-of-living adjustment riders?
- ❑ What's the best way to help protect my retirement income?
- ❑ When will a catastrophic disability benefit rider work in my favor?

Fig 5-2 Checklist of questions to ask when choosing a disability insurance policy.

Business Disability Insurance

Professional overhead expense insurance

Professional overhead expense insurance helps pay monthly business expenses, including rent, utilities, wages, and installment payments for business debt, as well as the costs associated with hiring a locum tenens (ie, temporary substitute) dentist. These policies have a benefit period of 1 to 2 years.

professional overhead expense insurance
Helps pay monthly business expenses, including rent, utilities, wages, and installment payments for business debt, as well as the costs associated with hiring a locum tenens (ie, temporary substitute) dentist.

Disability buyout policy

A disability buyout policy may be purchased for each partner in a practice who is eligible. If a partner becomes totally disabled, he or she is paid a benefit until "bought out." This occurs when the policy's maximum payment, based on a valuation of the company, has been paid; the disabled partner has recovered; or certain other conditions have been met.

disability buyout policy
Pays a benefit to a partner who has become totally disabled until he or she is "bought out" (ie, when the policy's maximum payment has been paid, the disabled partner has recovered, or certain other conditions have been met).

Business-reducing term insurance

Business-reducing term insurance is a type of disability insurance that pays fixed business obligations such as a loan, purchase agreement, or employment contract. However, most carriers do not offer this policy.

business-reducing term insurance
A type of disability insurance that pays fixed business obligations such as a loan, purchase agreement, or employment contract. Not offered by most carriers.

Choosing the Appropriate Disability Policy

A few important questions to ask an insurance adviser when choosing the appropriate disability policy for your situation are provided in the checklist in Fig 5-2.

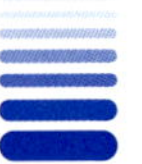

Before purchasing a policy, ask for a chance to review a proposal with the features and benefits you want, the premium amount, the base policy, and the cost of each additional rider. As a business owner, assess the risk of becoming sick or injured, then decide whether options such as overhead expense insurance, disability buyout insurance, or business-reducing term insurance are prudent given your age, health, responsibility, and future income.

Health Insurance

Having good health insurance and access to health care are major concerns, so the cost of health insurance premiums should be carefully weighed against proper coverage. Health care plans and rates vary between and within states, which can make it difficult to find the right plan for the individual, family, and employee. It's best to consult with an insurance adviser when choosing a health insurance plan because many factors may affect what type of plan is available. Certain things such as employment, health status, prior coverage, citizenship, and pre-existing conditions, as well as state laws, may help you decide what the proper coverage is for your situation. For the most part, full indemnity health insurance isn't a viable option because the cost of premiums for such plans is prohibitively high for the new dentist and employer, and sometimes it's not even available. The most common types of health care plans include the preferred provider organization (PPO), the health maintenance organization (HMO), and point-of-service (POS).

Preferred Provider Organization

preferred provider organization (PPO)
The insured chooses a physician and hospital for medical care from a list of preferred providers, a deductible is usually charged before the policy pays out, a copayment is sometimes charged for a covered service, and the total out-of-pocket expense is usually capped.

In most cases, the plan of choice is a PPO plan, in which the insured chooses a physician and hospital for medical care from a list of preferred providers. Each plan has its own particular features, but a deductible is usually charged before the policy pays out, and a copayment is sometimes charged for a covered service. However, the total out-of-pocket expense is usually capped.

Health Maintenance Organization

In some cases, an HMO plan is best. The out-of-pocket expense to the insured is less than that of a PPO because the choice of providers in the HMO network is more limited. An example of an HMO is Kaiser Permanente.

health maintenance organization (HMO)
Similar to a PPO, but the out-of-pocket expense to the insured is less because the choice of providers is more limited.

Point-of-Service

POS plans try to meld PPO access to providers with HMO cost, so that the insured chooses a primary care physician, who becomes the point-of-service and has an option to refer the insured out of network if needed.

point-of-service (POS)
The insured chooses a primary care physician, who becomes the point-of-service and has an option to refer the insured out of network if needed; considered a melding of PPO access to providers with HMO cost.

Health Savings Account

A unique health insurance option is the health savings account (HSA), which should be considered by every dentist, whether a recent graduate or long-time practitioner. You can make tax-deductible contributions to an HSA, then make withdrawals at any time tax-free to pay for qualified medical expenses. However, the catch is that an HSA must be coordinated with a high-deductible health insurance plan.

health savings account (HSA)
Account into which you can make tax-deductible contributions, then make withdrawals at any time tax-free to pay for qualified medical expenses. Must be coordinated with a high-deductible health insurance plan.

Health Insurance for Residents

Specialty and general practice residency (GPR) and Advanced Education in General Dentistry (AEGD) programs offer health insurance to residents. After the program is complete, the Consolidated Omnibus Reconciliation Act (COBRA) provides the opportunity for continuance of the health plan for up to 18 months, although the monthly premium, which may be higher than the original group rate, must be paid in full by the policyholder.

Employer-Paid Health Insurance

Employer-paid health insurance is an excellent benefit for employees, and group rates are usually lower than individual plans. Dental schools offer their faculty and families PPO, HMO, and POS plans. Independent contractors, however, don't qualify for employer-paid health plans.

An owner dentist has several options when offering health insurance to employees, including offering varying health insurance plans such as a PPO, HMO, or POS plan. As the owner dentist, you can choose to pay the premium for the employee or to pay a portion of the premium with the employee paying the difference. Some plans may be top heavy, where the owner has a higher-cost plan and the employee has a lower-cost plan, but not all plans allow this arrangement. Your accountant can provide guidance on the tax implications of providing health care insurance as an employer.

Health Insurance Offered by Dental Associations

Another way of obtaining health insurance is through a dental association, which may offer its members an array of health insurance plans. Other business and fraternal organizations may also offer group health plans to its members.

Life Insurance

Life insurance is issued either as a term policy or a permanent policy. A life insurance policy often features multiple riders, which add benefits to a policy.

Term Life Insurance

term life insurance
Pure insurance with no cash value or dividend and a limit on the length of the policy. Less expensive than permanent life insurance.

Term life insurance is pure insurance without cash value or dividend but with a limit on the length of the policy. Term life insurance is less expensive than permanent life insurance, and the premiums can be guaranteed not to increase for a period between 5 and 30 years. A premium is paid, and a beneficiary receives the face value upon the death of the insured. Policies are available up to age 70 or 80 years.

Permanent Life Insurance

permanent life insurance
Stays in force as long as the premium is paid and has cash value, which accrues as the policy matures and can be withdrawn as a loan (sometimes tax free).

Permanent life insurance is wholly different than term life insurance. Permanent life insurance stays in force for a lifetime–as long as the premium is paid. The policy has cash value, which accrues as the policy matures and can be withdrawn as a loan (sometimes tax free). Whole life, universal life, and variable life are three types of this insurance.

Whole life insurance

Whole life insurance has a fixed premium, with one portion allocated to a death benefit, usually in the form of a term life policy, and one portion that may build cash value.

whole life insurance
Type of permanent life insurance policy that has a fixed premium, with one portion allocated to a death benefit, usually in the form of a term life policy, and one portion that may build cash value.

Universal life insurance

Universal life insurance accrues cash value with greater flexibility to change the premium and death benefit compared with whole life insurance.

universal life insurance
Type of permanent life insurance policy that accrues cash value with greater flexibility to change the premium and death benefit compared with whole life insurance.

Variable life insurance

Variable life insurance is similar to universal life insurance. A variable policy allows you to invest its cash value into a mix of funds to meet your investment strategy (ie, the insured can invest the money into any of the funds the policy and carrier offers).

variable life insurance
Type of permanent life insurance policy that allows you to invest its cash value into a mix of funds to meet your investment strategy.

Life Insurance Terminology

Below is a list of common terminology related to life insurance policies, although different carriers may have variations of these terms that are specific to their products:

- *Death benefits:* Benefits paid to the named beneficiary upon the insured's death.
- *Face value:* The amount of the benefit stated in the policy.
- *Cash value:* The money that accrues in a permanent life insurance policy. There should be a guaranteed cash value and a projection based on current assumptions.
- *Dividend:* A percentage paid toward the cash value of a permanent policy. There is a guaranteed dividend and a current assumption.
- *Surrender value:* Cash value available in a permanent policy should that policy be cancelled.
- *Premium:* Cost of the insurance policy paid in monthly, quarterly, semiannual, or annual installments.
- *Rating:* Indication of quality of an insurance carrier as determined by a rating service.
- *Waiver of premium:* A rider that pays the policy premium in the event of a disability to the insured. The definition of a waiver of the premium varies among carriers.
- *Beneficiary:* The person(s) receiving the life insurance proceeds. A named beneficiary also can be a business, bank, or financial institution.

Uses for Life Insurance

Personal life insurance is intimately intertwined with the life and career of a dentist. Family protection is a paramount concern, and life insurance is a tool to cover expenses like mortgages, college education, and income to sustain a family in the event of death. It also can be used as an estate-planning tool because it pays the estate tax and forestalls premature liquidation of assets. In addition, the cash value of a permanent life insurance policy accumulates while the policy is in force, making it possible–up to a certain limit–to borrow against or withdraw from the cash accumulation on a tax-free basis.

Other uses for life insurance include:

- *Planning for personal and business purposes.* Life insurance needs constantly change throughout a career, so life events such as starting a practice, getting married, having children, and purchasing a home trigger the need for additional life insurance.
- *Private practice and business needs.* Banks and financial institutions may require that they be named as a beneficiary for the amount of a business loan in a life insurance policy. It's prudent to obtain a policy in the loan amount even if the financial institution doesn't require one.
- *Buy-sell stipulations in partnership agreements.* Partnership agreements have a mechanism in place to assign a value to the practice, which should be updated annually to reflect any increase or decrease. This is the amount one partner pays to purchase his or her share of the practice upon death or disability of the other partner. Life insurance benefits go to the estate to pay for the partnership share.
- *Key man insurance.* This is life insurance on a key partner, associate, employee, or insurable interest. For example, if a selling dentist is a key factor in the smooth transition of a practice for sale, life insurance on this individual would cover your loss should the seller not be available for full succession of the practice.
- *Real estate mortgage.* Life insurance can be used to cover the outstanding balance and allow your estate to cover this liability in the event of your death.

Conclusion

You should now be able to make an educated decision about the purchase of insurance for your personal and business life. The purchase of the proper insurance should not be something taken lightly, and policies should not be put away somewhere in a drawer or storage box to be forgotten. I learned about my policies and their shortcomings when it was too late to make any changes or additions, and my experiences with insurance as a disabled dentist led me on a crusade to educate health care professionals about insurance.

You spent years studying and investing hard work, time, and money to reach your goals, so make sure that you obtain the proper insurance to protect yourself, your business, and your family in the present and in the future.

Communicating Effectively in Dental Practice

Richard Nathan, DMD, MS

Following is a typical conversation heard at a 5-year dental school reunion:

> "It's the craziest feeling. It seems like it was only yesterday that we graduated and went off in all directions. Boy, I remember how scary that time was!"
>
> "Yeah, things worked out pretty well so far for most of the class."
>
> "For some more than others. Remember Michael? I mean, he was clinically average, certainly no G. V. Black. Well, I was talking to Charlie, who has a practice about a mile from Michael. It appears that our average-with-his-hands classmate's business is going gangbusters! Everyone in town ends up at Michael's practice. Charlie, who was arguably the best dentist in our class, is having a hard time getting business going. He's even lost patients to Michael! I don't get it."

Here are two dental practices that started up at the same time, with dentists who have identical training and who treat the same patient population. Yet, after 5 years, one is struggling to cover payroll and the other has a very busy and rewarding practice. So what would cause one dentist to do so much better than another?

There are, naturally, many possible explanations. A new dentist may overextend his or her practice with a big space, an extensive remodel, state-of-the art equipment, and a large staff. And, in too many instances, an excessive personal lifestyle may also play a part. Yet, the problem is not always overextension, bad luck, or poor decision making. In many cases it is the lack of a skill as important as clinical expertise that is not often taught in dental school. It's a skill everyone needs in order to facilitate personal and business relationships: effective communication.

Communicating with Patients

You may have exceptional clinical skills, but if you don't have the communication skills to establish trust with your patients, you'll never get the chance to use them.

If you can't communicate with your patients in a manner that motivates them to follow your treatment plan, the result is fewer patients on whom to practice your clinical skills. In other words, if you can't communicate, it doesn't matter how good of a dentist you are.

On the other hand, if you communicate with patients in a way that instills trust and confidence, they will talk glowingly about you at a cocktail party, the grocery store, and family affairs–people like to share the wealth. It's like finding a trusted car mechanic. Most people don't know what's going on under the hood of their car, so if they find someone they respect and who is honest with them, they will tell everyone they know about this gem. Trusting a dentist is even more important for most people than trusting a mechanic, yet the principle is the same. Patients spread the good word if they believe in you. However, if they think they're just another procedure in your schedule, they won't return, and they may even spread some not-so-good words.

Patients are excited to find a dentist they truly trust and want to spread the word to family, friends, and acquaintances.

Communicating with Your Staff

Staff members are seen by patients as an extension of you.

Successful communication doesn't just involve conversation with a patient. How you communicate with your employees and how they in turn communicate with your patients is also critical. Remember that each staff member is an extension of you. Both you and the staff must exude the kind of warmth and caring one extends when inviting a new friend to dinner.

Of course, hiring the right people is the first step in ensuring that you have a staff that communicates well. But, no less important is setting the right example with your words and actions. You are the captain of the ship. Believe it or not, your crew looks to you as a role model. Treat the staff and patients with the same respect and dignity that you expect when you are an employee or a patient.

Another reason to communicate well with your staff is that patients pay attention to how you treat your staff. Trust is lost when patients see a dentist acting one way with them and a very different way with the staff. Trust is hard to build but easy to lose, and verbally mistreating staff in front of a patient is one of the easiest ways to lose it.

Moreover, from a purely practical standpoint, staff members will leave you when you don't communicate effectively, empathically, and sincerely. No salary is high enough to compensate for being treated without dignity and respect. Remember how valuable your staff is–they perform important tasks that you don't want to perform or simply don't know how to perform–and treat them accordingly.

Three reasons to communicate well with your staff: (1) to set a good example, *(2)* to make a good impression on the patient, and *(3)* to improve staff retention.

The office is like the human body. Each organ has its own function. Yet, each organ is simultaneously dependent on the other organs for the whole system to function at peak performance. The staff is the lifeblood of the practice and the reason for its success. Don't take anyone on the staff for granted. Turnover is very costly for the employer and unsettling to your patients because they know that high turnover rates are a reflection of the dentist. Long-term staff is an indication of a boss who inspires and evokes loyalty, which will keep patients and attract new ones.

Listening

One of the fundamental aspects of developing effective communication skills is another ability for which dentists have little training–listening.

Listening to Understand

In *The 7 Habits of Highly Effective People,* Stephen R. Covey makes a cogent argument for the importance of listening with the intention of understanding.[1] This type of listening is the critical first step toward mutual understanding, trust, effective communication, and–ultimately–problem resolution.

Covey states that an essential principle is to "seek first to understand, then be understood."[1] This principle is analogous to the way in which we treat a patient. If a new patient walked into your office and complained that he'd had severe pain in the left mandible for 2 days, you wouldn't immediately pull out an elevator and forceps and extract his mandibular left third molar. What if the tooth could be saved with root canal or periodontal surgery? What if the pain is referred from a maxillary molar? Obviously, a radiograph is required, tooth vitality needs to be assessed, and periodontal probing should be performed before proper diagnosis, treatment, and prognosis can be determined. Dentists are trained to *diagnose first and then prescribe.*

Just as creating an effective treatment strategy is dependent upon fully understanding the patient's problem, being understood when you communicate is dependent upon understanding the perspective of the person with whom you are communicating.

Just as creating an effective treatment strategy is dependent upon fully understanding the patient's problem, being understood when you communicate is dependent upon understanding the perspective of the person with whom you are communicating. The vital element to understanding another person in professional and personal interactions is *listening.* Listening to understand means setting aside your wants and needs long enough to understand what the other person seeks from your interaction. Once the other person is allowed the space to open up and be heard, he or she is in a better place to understand much more of what you are saying, and you are better able to say what you need to say within the context of the other person's concerns and point of view.

Everyone needs to be heard. It's as basic a need as shelter, food, and love. When you take the time to listen and to "let your patients in," you initiate effective communication. It's about hearing the other person's story without filtering its meaning through your own lens. Becoming more receptive to what is said begins when you choose to "seek first to understand."[1] The ultimate goal is to be able to articulate and understand the other person's viewpoint as clearly as you can articulate and understand your own.

You must understand the patient's needs and desires before prescribing treatment if you want to gain compliance from the patient.

Two things happen when this is achieved. First, your original point of view will shift once you learn and understand the other person's perspective. Second, you gain trust and respect and, thus, become more influential. This is critical to any case presentation. You must understand the patient's needs and desires before prescribing treatment if you want to gain compliance from the patient.

Listening to understand is critical to any situation in which communication and, particularly, conflict resolution is required, whether it is with a patient, staff, other health care professionals, or the larger world outside the office–colleagues, specialist referrals, dental technicians, supply representatives, financial officers, dental school faculty, or local businesses.

Establishing Trust and Mutual Understanding

If you really listen to patients during an initial consultation and let them explain their situation, they will sense that you respect who they are and what they need, and they will begin to trust you.

Attentive body language is a function of effective listening. Body language sends strong nonverbal signals of interest, and there are many gestures or cues that suggest empathy and result in reciprocal attention. Conversely, unfocused body and eye movements project a sense of distraction. As you listen to a patient, be still with a fixed gaze that sends the message that you care and don't want to miss a word. An open body stance with unfolded arms conveys a sense of being mentally open to what is being said, and leaning slightly forward toward the speaker conveys interest in what is being said. Be patient. Don't interrupt. Give space to expand. Listen until the thought is fully finished, even if you are eager to interrupt. There are always competing distractions in the office such as phone calls, but make it a policy never to be interrupted when you are with a patient. Show that you are only interested in the patient at that time.

Body language sends strong nonverbal signals of interest, and there are many gestures or cues that suggest empathy and result in reciprocal attention. Conversely, unfocused body and eye movements project a sense of distraction.

Being a good listener is not easy. I remember a case presentation I mismanaged at the beginning of my career. A new patient came in for a consultation, and, after reviewing the radiographs and clinical readings, I presented a detailed explanation of the problem and treatment plan to the patient.

> "Well, Mr Smith," I began confidently, "it appears from my extensive examination that you have generalized severe periodontal disease that has caused many of your teeth to become loose. In fact, some of your teeth have to be extracted. I noticed from your dental history form that you haven't been to a dentist in more than 10 years, which, of course, is why the situation in your mouth has deteriorated so severely. Well, that's water under the bridge now, isn't it? What's important is that we start right away to get you back in shape with periodontal surgery. I'll add artificial bone under your gums in order to reestablish support around the teeth that have lost bone. We'll extract the bad teeth at that time. Once healed, we'll send you back to your general dentist for restorative work. As we progress with the work, I'll fill you in with more details. So, do you have any questions for me at this time?"
>
> "No."
>
> "Well, then, why don't you go out front and make the first appointment? We can get started getting your mouth back in shape as soon as possible."

After making an appointment for the first dental surgery, Mr Smith said goodbye and left the office. In fact, he left for good. He never showed up for the appointment, and I never saw him again. I did hear about him, though, about 2 years later, after receiving a phone call from one of my professors. Mr Smith had presented with an abscess in the emergency clinic at the dental school where I was trained. He was seen by an attending periodontist who had been on faculty when I was a resident.

After Mr Smith was relieved of the acute problem, the periodontist asked when he last saw a dentist and why periodontal treatment was never completed. Mr Smith told him that he had seen me for a consultation visit 2 years before but didn't follow up with the prescribed treatment. Since this dentist was willing to listen, Mr Smith told his version of what I had done to scare him away.

It turns out that Mr Smith had gone through a rather traumatic dental experience 10 years before he came to see me that had left him incapable of trusting what I had to say. He was unable to resolve the negative effect associated with the past event, so I effectively negated my ability to gain his trust by failing to provide him the space and time to tell his story. I was too caught up in my own story and the obvious clinical necessity of the treatment plan I proposed. I established neither trust nor credibility because I didn't take the time to listen and understand him. All I needed to do was to give him the chance to express his concern about his past experiences. If he had felt confidence in my ability and willingness to listen, then the barrier between his emotions and what I was saying would have dissipated. Seeking to understand, I would have been understood.

I established neither trust nor credibility because I didn't take the time to listen and understand him. All I needed to do was to give him thc chancc to express his concern about his past experiences. If he had felt confidence in my ability and willingness to listen, then the barrier between his emotions and what I was saying would have dissipated.

Let's imagine what might have been a much more productive encounter:

"So, Mr Smith, let me show you your mouth on the radiographs. Here's my areas of concern on the tooth model."

"Okay, but I've been told by another periodontist that I had severe gum disease."

"Oh, really? When was that?"

"Well, it was about 10 years ago."

"So, what happened? Did he do any treatment?"

"Well, not really. I went in for a consultation, and he immediately scheduled me for full-mouth surgery that very afternoon! He said my case was extremely bad, and I shouldn't put off treatment. My head was spinning. I didn't quite understand why I was seeing a periodontist and not my general dentist who referred me. I didn't really have any pain to speak of. Then, all of a sudden, I'm about to have all my gums opened up, teeth extracted, and bone grafted."

"Wow! That must have been traumatic."

"Yeah, no kidding! But that wasn't the worst part. When I hesitated to schedule treatment that afternoon, the periodontist got really upset with me. He told me that he had seen hundreds of cases like mine, and he knew what was best for me. He said that I was in denial of the obvious. Patients like me wind up losing their teeth within a short period of time."

"What did you say then?"

"I said, 'Goodbye!'"

"Okay. Well, let's proceed slowly, one step at a time. First, tell me what you know about the condition of your mouth. I want to know what you know and how you feel about being here."

"Thank you. Really, thank you very much. I truly appreciate the fact that you are open to hear my point of view."

In this scenario, we listened to each other and developed mutual understanding and trust, which put us in a position to begin a real conversation. Mr Smith was now open to a logical discussion about the current state of his mouth and what we could accomplish through treatment, creating the possibility of reaching a mutually agreed-upon solution. He was more likely to feel like he was part of the process, involved in the therapy, and therefore more committed to the result.

As this example illustrates, in order to realize the desired result, we must begin with effective listening, which will hopefully lead to mutual understanding and trust and, ultimately, effective communication.

Taking the Initial Phone Call

As stated before, in the eyes of your patients, your staff members are an extension of yourself. What they say and do reflects directly on you. The initial phone contact with a new patient is critical to success. Your staff should "smile" through the phone. True, a caller can't see the smile, but a caller can surely feel its warmth. It gives a sense of welcome. Patients should feel that the entire office staff is looking forward to meeting them and making their appointment comfortable. If possible, an initial caller should never be put on hold. If a staff member must put a caller on hold, he or she should apologize sincerely, ask the caller's permission to place him or her on hold, wait for a response, then let the caller know that the call will be returned to as soon as possible.

Patients should feel that the entire office staff is looking forward to meeting them and making their appointment comfortable.

Staff should be trained to be patient with new patients. The process is new to them, and they need to ask many questions. In difficult economic times, patients want to know the price of the examination and cleaning. They want to know if their insurance is accepted and what treatments their insurance will cover. Staff will need to explain your insurance policy and the estimated deductible and copayment. If staff does not have immediate access to the patient's specific insurance information, he or she should assure the patient that by the first visit the insurance coverage will be researched and the benefits explained.

It's important during the initial call that a new patient is given the opportunity to express any fears and apprehension he or she may have about a dental visit.

It's important during the initial call that a new patient is given the opportunity to express any fears and apprehension he or she may have about a dental visit. In other words, staff must exercise the skill of listening to understand by giving the patient the space and time to express any concerns. A simple explanation can allay many fears. At the very least, it will let the new patient know that you and your staff care. It's simple, really. We all have been patients, so make sure that you and your staff treat a new patient with the same respect and dignity that you would expect if you were in the same place. New patients who feel valued become loyal patients in the future.

Creating a Good First Impression

Office Décor

Your office sends subtle messages about you to every new patient through its décor, lighting, selected reading materials, and cleanliness.

Your office sends subtle messages about you to every new patient through its décor, lighting, selected reading materials, and cleanliness. Whether it is comfortable and casual or high-end glitz, make sure that your office décor accurately represents the image you want to project.

Magazine selection is always a topic of discussion at my office. Should we keep getting *Sports Illustrated*? What about *Reader's Digest* this year? An eclectic assortment of light reading with news, business, entertainment, sports, and women's topics should probably be represented, then supplemented with periodicals that make a statement about the dentist's personal interests like health, fitness, tennis, golf, or even parenting.

From the first day of practice, I had a professional photo of my two daughters when they were 2 years and 5 years of age nicely framed for my waiting room. Over the years, I added more photos of the girls as they grew up and a few of the whole family in my operatories. Patients have always commented favorably about the photos. My experience is that images of you and your family–even your pets–are an important part of the office décor because they inspire feelings of comfort and trust in your patients.

Staff Greeting

How your staff communicates with the new patient is even more critical than what is on the walls. Despite being busy, the staff must check the day sheet to know when a new patient is expected and should be present to greet the patient with a smile and identify him or her by name. The staff should also assist patients who require help filling out the medical history and insurance forms.

Staff should be aware of the upcoming arrival of any new patients and greet them by name in a warm and friendly manner.

Language assistance may be critical in certain locations. My staff is multilingual. Chinese, Spanish, and Russian are spoken in addition to English. Being able to communicate in the patient's native language is one more step toward developing a trusting relationship, and the ease of a multilingual office can be invaluable for promoting referrals.

Initial Examination and Case Presentation

Your first opportunity to use effective communication skills is in the initial examination. Remember that your mantra is, "Seek first to understand, then to be understood."[1] Listen carefully to build mutual understanding and trust. Follow with a straightforward discussion of the patient's concerns and problems. Keep in mind that needs (logical) and wants (emotional) aren't necessarily the same. Use clinical skills to determine needs and communication skills to determine wants. An ethical and successful dentist never attempts to "sell a case." The dentist doesn't preach; instead, the dentist *educates* and presents the patient with a *solution* based on his or her needs and wants.

An ethical and successful dentist never attempts to "sell a case," but rather educates the patient and presents a solution based on his or her needs and wants.

Every new patient is valuable. The two categories of patients in a practice are new and recall patients. The new patient produces between four to five times more for the practice than a recall patient. Compared with the existing recall patient, this patient is more likely to refer other new patients.

New patients are more likely than existing recall patients to refer other new patients, making them valuable assets who should be treated with special care and respect.

Opening Dialogue

The first impression is the most lasting. The first thing I do when I meet a new patient is to sit at eye level and say, "Hello, Mr Smith. My name is Richard Nathan. I'm very glad to meet you. So, what brings you here today?" This salutation brings up two issues. The first consideration is what to call yourself when addressing a patient. For me, should it be "Dr Nathan," "Richard Nathan," or just "Richard"? This is an individual decision, but I have my own parameters when making this determination. I am "Dr Nathan" to patients who are 24 years of age and younger. Patients in this age group are more comfortable with a formal relationship. To other patients, I am "Richard Nathan" most of the time. Interestingly, some patients who have been with me for 30 years still call me Dr Nathan! Perhaps these patients feel comfortable maintaining professional distance.

By asking patients what has brought them into the office, I invite them into the process and give them the chance to express any wants or needs. It reminds me not to preach to the patient but rather to allow the conversation to begin with the patient's concern. The patient might say, "I'm here because I think I lost a filling," or, "I haven't been to the dentist for 10 years." Generally, patients don't know what's going on inside their mouths. You aren't asking the question to help with the overall diagnosis; you ask to show that you care and respect the patient's opinion. The introductory question opens up a dialogue and creates an opportunity to establish a working alliance.

The introductory question opens up a dialogue and creates an opportunity to establish a working alliance.

Building the Dentist-Patient Relationship

When you present a treatment plan, it is important to be realistic and truthful.

Building a thriving and prosperous practice is all about building successful relationships one patient at a time. Remember that relationships are based on trust, and building trust begins with telling the truth, so when you present a treatment plan, it is important to be realistic and truthful. Being realistic about a prognosis is a clinical judgment call; yet, in order to retain trust, it is important for the dentist and the patient to have similar expectations of what the future brings. Expectations should be presented in a manner that is easily understood and clearly documented in the chart.

Speak to patients in plain English without dental jargon. Don't be afraid to repeat important concepts during a case presentation, and give the patient plenty of opportunities to ask questions.

Patients are not impressed with multisyllabic words, so speak in plain English without dental jargon. Don't be afraid to repeat important concepts twice or even three times during a case presentation. There is a lot of information for the patient to absorb at one time. An anxious patient may be too overwhelmed to fully understand what is being said; therefore, it's helpful if you give the patient multiple opportunities to ask questions.

While diagnosing the patient's dental issue at the initial examination, carefully listen to understand the patient's motivation. Some people are motivated to retain natural teeth in a disease-free state, some are driven by esthetics, and others are financially constrained and interested in value over time or simply the least expensive alternative. Most patients are motivated by a combination of these factors. Let's say that a patient has recurrent decay around an old filling and that a full-coverage crown is the best treatment. If you determine that this patient is finance or value oriented, you might explain the long-term value of a crown restoration compared with a large amalgam.

While making a diagnosis at the initial examination, carefully listen to understand the patient's motivation: retaining natural teeth, esthetics, long-term value, the least expensive alternative, or a combination of these.

Visual aids are an important means of effective communication during the initial examination. If the patient is given a handheld mirror, he or she can follow the clinical examination. Then the findings can be further explained through radiographs, a tooth model, a photograph, or a diagram. Intraoral camera images shown in real time on a large monitor can be used with great effectiveness. Patients integrate new concepts in different ways, so it's good to cover every angle. Some learn best by what they hear during the presentation, while others learn best visually through radiographs, models, images, and diagrams.

Some patients learn better by listening, while others find visual information easier to process, so cover all of your bases by both telling and showing the patient what needs to be done.

Finally, there are times when you must tell a patient that you are not able to help. The dentist develops the ability and skill to deliver a variety of services and treatment, but he or she must also have the integrity to say, "I do not have the capability to meet your needs." In these cases, a patient is grateful for your honesty and is likely to follow through with a referral to a specialist.

Be honest with patients about the limits of your expertise and training and refer to specialists when needed.

Emergency Treatment Visits

Many times the first new patient appointment is an emergency visit. The patient may be in pain and seeking immediate relief, so be sure to communicate to the patient that you are confident in your ability to address the problem and set aside time to do so. Focus only on the immediate issue at hand during an emergency appointment. Diagnose the presenting problem and deliver the needed treatment; save any discussion of a comprehensive treatment plan for another appointment; and resist the temptation to place blame on lack of oral hygiene and failure to make regular dental visits. If the problem requires a specialist, have your front desk call the specialist's office, emphasize the emergency nature of the problem, then schedule the first available time for the patient. Call another specialist if the first specialist cannot see the patient immediately. At the very least, deliver infection and pain management treatment to alleviate the symptoms until the specialist can see the patient, then call the patient later that evening or the next day to check on his or her status.

Treating emergencies is a great way to build your practice.

Treating emergencies is a great way to build your practice. New dentists can sign up with the local dental society, hospital emergency room, and hotel concierge to serve as a dental emergency resource. Many of my most loyal and best referring patients began years ago as emergency visits.

Honesty About Pain

You'll lose a child's trust if you tell him or her that something won't hurt at all and it does, even if it's just a little pain.

The issue of discomfort during dental treatment should be addressed honestly with all patients, but especially with children. When giving injections, tell a child that it hurts only for a moment when he or she is first injected, and then the area becomes numb or feels fat. Then explain that the child will feel pressure after the injection but no sharp pain. You'll lose a child's trust if you tell him or her that it won't hurt at all and it does, even if it's just a little pain. Painless injection is a skill that is acquired, so provide topical, warm anesthetic and a light touch. However, there are times when it's impossible to give a painless injection, such as when giving a palatal injection, so let the patient know that care will be taken to make sure the injection procedure is as gentle and comfortable as possible.

Unnecessary Communication

Never chat with a chairside assistant about unrelated topics when treating a patient. The patient in the chair expects your undivided attention to be on his or her treatment.

There are times when talking is not warranted. Never–and I mean *never*–chat with a chairside assistant about unrelated topics when treating a patient. The patient in the chair expects your undivided attention to be on his or her treatment. Conversation should be limited to essential issues regarding the current procedure. There's plenty of time for friendly chatter with the patient and staff before and after the dental treatment–but not during any procedures.

A dentist can be too attentive during dental procedures. Patients generally do not want you to ask them every 2 minutes how they're doing or if they're all right. This is annoying and leads them to suspect that you aren't confident about the treatment's progress. Occasionally, I ask patients if they are okay and if they need to rest their jaw muscles. Patients usually want to get the procedure completed in a timely manner, so get in and get out efficiently.

The Angry Patient

There are times when you must deal with an upset and angry patient. Some new patients come to the office with a chip on their shoulder about an injustice endured at the hands of another dentist. The first words out of their mouths are a diatribe about a substandard crown that doesn't feel right, severe pain during a root canal, or the dentist's foul breath and body odor. However tempting it may be, do not collude in the criticism of another dentist.

Let the patient vent feelings, then offer an empathic yet firm comment: "I'm very sorry you had difficulty in the past, but let's see what your current dental problems are and see what I can do to help." By criticizing others in the profession, we criticize ourselves. Even when we observe subpar dentistry, we understand that untoward outcomes occur and are sometimes uncontrollable.

The more difficult situation is when the patient is upset with you. You may make a mistake in diagnosis and treatment or convey unrealistic expectations to patients. Dental practice isn't a perfect science. Sometimes the human body, procedure, or dental material just doesn't cooperate. Expect to be challenged by patients throughout your career. Patient anger and complaints may or may not be justified. Your response should be the same regardless of the situation. Do not become defensive. Implement the cardinal rule of effective communication: Stop and listen empathically. Begin to build trust by first attempting to understand the patient's point of view, then explaining your perspective. Speak to the patient in a calm and caring manner in order to reach a mutually agreeable solution.

Dental practice isn't a perfect science. Expect to be challenged by patients throughout your career.

Conclusion

Successful communication in dentistry boils down to a very simple concept: *effective listening*. If you learn how to listen to patients, staff, colleagues, and business partners, you'll be surprised at how pleasurable the daily operation of your office becomes. All parties will be satisfied and enthusiastic in an environment that generally results in a productive and prosperous practice. Trust me. I'm listening.

Reference

1. Covey SR. The 7 Habits of Highly Effective People, ed 15. New York: Simon and Schuster, 2004.

Understanding Basic Finances

Michael Okuji, DDS, MPH, MBA

This chapter introduces basic finance, accounting, and tax concepts. No previous finance knowledge is necessary to grasp the principles presented. The goal is to make you sufficiently conversant to engage advisers and to make business decisions in an environment of uncertainty. Financial acumen is just as important to the success of a dental practice as clinical expertise. As a dentist, you must take and keep control of cash flow and use good judgment in tandem with maintaining accurate records and defined controls. Finance (a judicious use of loans, cash flow control, and consistent income) converts your intangible assets (your dental degree, skill, time, and energy) into tangible asset capital (home and property equity, investment accounts, and retirement funds) over time.

Financial acumen is just as important to the success of a dental practice as clinical expertise.

It is true that dentists who started private practice decades ago were able to become financially secure without the benefit of business training in or out of dental school. During that period of time, there was rapid population growth and widespread indemnity insurance. That meant that dentists could increase production from a new population of patients who had recently acquired indemnity insurance, then raise their fees in an unregulated market. The invisible hand of the market didn't modulate demand or price, and the unimpeded cash influx ameliorated inefficient business practice and wasteful management decisions. However, this isn't

In today's dental business world, when office overhead shoots through the roof, any business inefficiency is magnified, and there is very little room for error.

the case today; instead, managed care contracts limit fees, even though office expenses continue to rise and regulatory mandates on dental business operations become more incursive. So, when office overhead shoots through the roof, any business inefficiency is magnified, and there is very little room for error.

It isn't practical for dental schools to introduce more business management hours into the curriculum. Dental students don't need a master of business administration degree and, more importantly, they don't have the time in an already overcrowded curriculum. Instead, students just need the basic tools that will allow them to understand the concepts and vocabulary of business so they can ask the appropriate questions and become demanding consumers of professional advice.

Each of the sections in the chapter introduces a basic finance concept and is written for the dentist who has no experience in business and does not have a family member in business or dentistry.

Business System

Every dental practice requires a business system that will guide major and minor management decisions, such as the purchase of dental equipment and ordering supplies. All decisions impact the finances of the practice. Some dentists manage on an ad hoc basis and react and interact only when there isn't enough money in the checking account to meet the payroll or pay the laboratory, but the prudent dentist operates as a manager who continually tracks and analyzes key financial indicators of the practice to maintain a smooth system that will anticipate economic downturns. The business system itself is divided into investment, finance, and operation decisions.

The prudent dentist operates as a manager who continually tracks and analyzes key financial indicators of the practice to maintain a smooth system that will anticipate economic downturns.

Investment Decisions

Investment decisions provide funds to purchase new equipment and facilities and fund spending plans, such as advertising and promotion, to support the vision of the practice. The key question in an investment decision is its return, for example: What is the expected revenue and net income generated from an in-office dental ceramic milling machine over its lifetime?

The key question in an investment decision is its return.

Finance Decisions

Finance decisions involve selecting the relative proportion of funds from borrowed money (debt obligations) and internal sources (retained earnings) to fuel the investment. Will the financial leverage from borrowed money to purchase the in-office ceramic milling machine return more income than the cost of its operation, principal, and interest? Can this same borrowed money or internal cash be better spent on another investment, such as an intraoral camera or an electric handpiece?

Finance decisions involve selecting the relative proportion of funds from borrowed money (debt obligations) and internal sources (retained earnings) to fuel the investment.

Operation Decisions

An operation decision is characterized as the use of net dental income to provide further services to patients. Operational fund allocation is a tradeoff between the pricing of procedures and their cost effectiveness. Will the fee and time saved by a milled crown offset the cost of the space, maintenance, supplies, training, and staff that it requires? Will patients readily see the value of the same-day procedure? In other words, will it enhance internal marketing and increase demand and new patient flow?

Operational fund allocation is a tradeoff between the pricing of procedures and their cost effectiveness.

Another example of an operation decision is whether treating a new group of managed care patients within a preferred provider organization (PPO) with the existing staff is efficient or whether more staff members will be required. Does the new PPO patient inflow and PPO fee sufficiently offset the higher operating cost, thus resulting in more net income?

Time Value of Money

A dollar in your pocket today is worth more than a dollar collected tomorrow. This is called the time value of money. It is a concept that is used every day. It is applied when purchasing an existing practice, buying new equipment, or developing a collection philosophy. What will the money invested or spent today on a piece of equipment, extending credit to patients, or on another investment be worth tomorrow in today's dollar? This is the present value of an investment. The present value of future expected earnings is determined using discounted cash flow (DCF). Its name is derived from the fact that it uses a discount rate to calculate the present dollar value of expected future cash flow.

In the time value of money, the converse of present value is future value. Present value calculates the value of tomorrow's collection today,

time value of money
A dollar in your pocket today is worth more than a dollar collected tomorrow.

present value
Calculation of the value of tomorrow's collection today using a discount.

discounted cash flow (DCF)
Calculation of the present dollar value of expected future cash flow with an appropriate discount rate.

future value
Calculation of the value of today's collection tomorrow using a compound rate.

while future value calculates the value of today's collection tomorrow. To do so, it uses a compound rate. The time interval used for discounting and compounding can be annual, semiannual, quarterly, weekly, daily, or overnight in certain central bank transactions. A more frequent discount or compound interval results in a higher cost of funds or return on funds.

One useful present value calculation for a family is to estimate the number of dollars that must be invested today to pay for a newborn child's college tuition in 18 years. The DCF formula calculates the present value of expected future cash flows and is expressed as:

$$\$ = \sum \frac{¢}{(1+r)^{t1}} + \frac{¢}{(1+r)^{t2}} + \frac{¢}{(1+r)^{t3}} \quad . . .$$

The present value (\$) equals the sum (Σ) of expected future cash flow (¢) divided by 1 + discount rate (r) at a time (t) expressed in years, ie, $t1 = 1$ year, $t2 = 2$ years, $t3 = 3$ years, etc.

It is a relatively easy formula to use–just plug in the appropriate numbers. That's the science. The art is choosing the appropriate numbers. In all financial forecasts, DCF requires estimates based on uncertainty. The discount rate is usually selected based on other investments of a similar nature with the same level of risk. It takes into account all investment factors, including expectations, risk, time frame, and financial leverage (debt).

opportunity cost of capital
Another name for the discount rate. Its name is derived from the fact that it represents the rate of return that could be earned by investing in the next best alternative.

The discount rate is also called the opportunity cost of capital because it is an estimate of the rate of return an investor would receive in another venture of similar risk (ie, the foregone opportunity). An expected cash flow over 5 years from a practice with an unstable patient base carries a higher risk and a higher discount rate (perhaps based on returns from a high-risk investment like drilling an oil well) than a similar practice with a solid base of patients (with a discount rate selected based on the rate of return on a low-risk investment like a treasury bond).

Valuation

Because dental practice is still a cottage industry, there is no continuous large market of buyers and sellers who submit financial reports using generally accepted accounting principles (GAAP) under the scrutiny of the US Securities and Exchange Commission (SEC) with stock prices published daily. Therefore, it is important that you, as a new dentist, are able

Box 7-1 Calculations to determine expected net free cash flow

	Revenue
–	Office expense
+	Discretionary expense
	Operating income
+	Depreciation and amortization
+	Loan interest and principal
	Net operating income
–	Dentist salary
	Net free cash flow

to perform a valuation of your own practice or on an existing practice you are considering for purchase.

Goodwill

Present value

As mentioned in chapter 3, future cash flow is an intangible asset called *goodwill* that is purchased with a practice and is probably the only reason to buy an existing practice. A buyer's principal goal when purchasing an existing dental practice is to determine the present value of the expected future cash flow of the practice.

Calculating net free cash flow

The first step in finding the present value of expected future cash flow is to determine the expected net free cash flow. The basic formula for calculating net free cash flow is shown in Box 7-1.

Begin by looking at the practice's historical operating income, which is the cash left after deducting only those expenses directly associated with the operation of the practice. To accomplish this, after deducting office expenses, you'll need to add back any included discretionary expenses, ie, unique, elective expenditures that the present owner incurred, such as travel to Hawaii for a dental convention. You can simplify this process by creating a spreadsheet that will verify operating income based on past performance. Cross check the previous dentist's bank statement revenue and expense categories against the Schedule C income tax return categories for the same year (see chapter 8), then verify each reported revenue and

net free cash flow
Cash available to a practice after deducting operating expenses and a reasonable dentist's salary. Used to calculate expected future cash flow.

operating income
Cash left after deducting only those expenses directly associated with the operation of the practice.

expense category over a 3- to 5-year interval. The federal income tax return Schedule C revenue and expense numbers don't always mirror the bank statement; in these cases the bank statement should be taken as the correct source for both revenue and expense.

depreciation
Gradual conversion of the cost of a tangible asset into an expense over the estimated useful life of the asset.

amortization ***(def 1)***
Gradual conversion of the cost of an intangible asset into an expense over the estimated useful life of the asset.

Add back depreciation and amortization, the noncash, tax-deduction entries that may be listed on Schedule C but not the bank statement. These are only accounting entries, not checkbook entries, ie, they don't affect cash flow. Then, add back loan interest and principal payments because they, as well as depreciation and amortization, are financing and investment transactions not related to the direct operation of the practice. The final spreadsheet tabulation should now show revenue, expense, and net operating income for 3 to 5 years. Ask yourself whether the annual numbers in each category decline, remain level, or rise over this period. Is the total practice income growing, stable, or in decline? Did the owner "pad" the net operating income by increasing production in the year prior to the sale to make the practice net income look better? Did the increased production deplete future treatment in the present patient base while not adding any new patients? These last two questions are "qualitative" practice valuation issues that don't appear on a bank statement or income tax return.

net operating income
Operating income after financial noncash expenses (eg, depreciation and amortization) are added back.

One way to attempt to determine the quality of the net operating income figure is by inspecting a sample of patient charts to gauge their longevity in the practice, recent treatment activity, future treatment needs, and referral history. You can also look at the appointment book for new patient appointments, broken appointments, slow periods, and the number of vacation days and holidays taken, then analyze the financial ledger to calculate accounts receivable that are 30 days, 60 days, and more than 60 days outstanding; the turnover rate (ie, time interval between production and collection of revenue from patient services); the amount of bad debt; and the managed care fee write-offs.

turnover rate
Time interval between production and collection of revenue from patient services.

bad debt
Accounts receivable that are more than 120 days past due and thus considered uncollectible.

Another consideration is that the imputed present value of the expected cash flow is weakened by the recent general incursion of managed care dental plans into dental practice because of their stipulated lower fees. Patients become loyal to the managed care plan or an organized union sponsor rather than to the dentist. Moreover, in all dental practice purchases, a certain percentage of patient attrition can be expected for a number of intrinsic and extrinsic reasons. This lack of stability in the patient base can be accounted for by deducting a percentage from the net operating income figure.

Box 7-2 Calculations to determine the net free cash flow of a simplified hypothetical practice

Revenue		**$500,000**
Office expense	–	$300,000
Discretionary expense	+	$0
Operating income		**$200,000**
Depreciation and amortization	+	$0
Loan interest and principal paid	+	$0
Net operating income		**$200,000**
Dentist salary	–	$150,000
Net free cash flow		**$50,000**

Finally, deduct a reasonable dentist salary from the net operating income. For this figure you might infer the wage that the dentist could earn outside of the practice as a full-time employee elsewhere. Deducting the salary from a clean net operating income gives the expected net free cash flow number from which you compute the present value of future cash flow.

The dentist salary deducted from net operating income to get net free cash flow is based on the wages that the dentist could earn outside of the practice as a full-time employee elsewhere.

As an example, let's calculate the net free cash flow of a simplified hypothetical practice that produces $500,000 gross revenue with $300,000 operating expense, no personal expense deduction, and zero attrition (Box 7-2). The operating income is calculated to be $200,000 and, assuming the buyer can earn $150,000 as a full-time associate outside of the practice, $50,000 is left as the net free cash flow.

Calculating present value of expected future cash flow

Continuing the example from the previous section, if net free cash flow is expected to be $50,000 each year, then what is this steady cash stream worth today? In other words, what is its present value?

There are two variables to consider when estimating the present value of future cash flow: *(1)* the appropriate discount rate (a zero discount rate infers no risk, no inflation, and no time value of money) and *(2)* the time period, which is usually considered to be when a new practice startup can earn the same free cash flow as the purchased practice. However, both variables are uncertain, best-guess assumptions that the buyer and seller will most likely disagrcc on. Noticc that thc futurc cffort of thc pur chasing dentist to increase practice efficiency, production, and net income are not variables in the present value calculation because that value is added to the practice by the purchasing dentist's efforts alone and is not attributed to the previous dentist.

The DCF formula below shows that the present value of a steady annual stream of $50,000 in expected future cash flow derived from goodwill only over a 3-year period at a 4.0% discount rate is $138,755.

$$\$138{,}755 = \sum \frac{\$50{,}000}{(1.04)^1} + \frac{\$50{,}000}{(1.04)^2} + \frac{\$50{,}000}{(1.04)^3}$$

Table 7-1 shows the present value of $50,000 calculated using DCF at three different discount rates. If you were considering purchasing this practice, you'd have to ask yourself a few questions, such as: In this analysis, does $50,000 annual free cash flow sound right? Is there an attrition factor? Would you pay $150,000 today for the expected $50,000 annual cash flow over a 3-year period with some money not collected for 3 years? If not, would you pay $138,755 today for an expected $50,000 annual free cash flow over the next 3 years?

Maybe you think the expected cash flow is risky because of the number of managed care patients in the practice, so you use a 12.5% discount rate instead. The present value of the 3-year annual free cash flow is now $119,067, or about $20,000 less (see Table 7-1). Does this make more sense for this particular practice? Is paying an additional $20,000 to $30,000 a deal breaker for you or the seller? Finally, is the expected free cash flow sufficient to repay the practice loan?

You might feel that starting a new practice in a tight economy infused with managed care plans and building it to a level of $50,000 annual free cash flow will take 5 instead of 3 years. In this case, you would calculate the present value over that 5-year period (Table 7-2). Now the difference between the high and low present values is more than $70,000. You would have to ask yourself what value makes sense and whether the valuation difference is going to be a deal breaker between yourself and the seller.

Determining net present value

net present value (NPV) The present value of the expected future free cash flow minus the initial cost of the investment. A positive NPV suggests that an investment will provide a good return.

In finance, net present value (NPV) measures the free cash flow of the future cash benefits against the current investment, which allows the buyer to determine whether the net balance between present value and practice cost is favorable or not. Algebraically, NPV equals the present value of the expected future free cash flow *less* the initial cost of the investment (ie, selling price of the practice). If the NPV is positive, then it may be a good investment, but if the NPV is negative, then the opposite may be

Table 7-1 Present value of $50,000 over 3 years using DCF at three discount rates

Discount (%)	Year 1 ($)	Year 2 ($)	Year 3 ($)	Present value ($)
0.0	50,000	50,000	50,000	150,000
4.0	48,077	46,228	44,450	138,755
12.5	44,444	39,506	35,117	119,067

Table 7-2 Present value of $50,000 over 5 years using DCF at three discount rates

Discount (%)	Year 1 ($)	Year 2 ($)	Year 3 ($)	Year 4 ($)	Year 5 ($)	Present value ($)
0.0	50,000	50,000	50,000	50,000	50,000	250,000
4.0	48,077	46,228	44,450	42,740	41,096	222,591
12.5	44,444	39,506	35,117	31,215	27,746	178,028

true. For example, if the present value of the expected future free cash flow is $178,028 and the practice sales price for goodwill is $175,000, the NPV is positive, so one is inclined to make the investment. Alternatively, if the sales price for goodwill is $180,00, the NPV is negative, and one is disinclined to make the deal.

Payback period

A payback period is another method for valuing the goodwill of a dental practice. It estimates the number of years it takes to pay back the original investment and is a quick way to determine whether the investment can be repaid within its economic life. In other words, it tells you whether the capability of the practice meets its financial obligation to pay back the practice loan. Algebraically, payback equals the cost of investment divided by the expected annual free cash flow per year (not adjusted for the time value of money).

payback period
The amount of time it takes to pay back the original investment, calculated as the cost of investment divided by the expected annual free cash flow per year. Used to determine whether the investment can be repaid within its economic life.

Present value and payback are similar, but the major difference between them is that present value builds in an earnings requirement in addition to recovering the initial investment. This is a critical concept to grasp because the goal of a business enterprise is to maximize its return on investment, not just to break even. So, to settle on a purchase price that simply breaks even is not sufficient reason to invest in a particular practice when other practice opportunities of similar nature and risk are available.

To settle on a purchase price that simply breaks even is not sufficient reason to invest in a particular prac tice when other practice opportunities of similar nature and risk are available.

Profitability index

profitability index
Present value of expected future cash flow divided by the price of the practice.

Two practices may have identical present value expectations but different size revenue streams and different required investments (ie, prices), so their respective profitability index is different. The profitability index is equal to the present value of expected future cash flow divided by the price of the practice. Generally speaking, for the buyer, the higher the profitability index, the better. However, in some cases there may be intrinsic qualitative features that would justify the purchase of a practice with a lower profitability index.

Final analysis

Valuation of goodwill is a voodoo art. Purchasing an intangible asset is fraught with ambiguity and uncertainty, and the buyer and seller are destined to disagree on all aspects of the valuation. What is the expected future cash flow, including operating income, leading to free cash flow? What is the appropriate discount rate to apply, and what is the number of years to consider? However, in the final analysis, the practice value is the amount a buyer is willing to pay and a seller is willing to accept. Nothing else matters.

Ultimately, the value of a practice is the amount a buyer is willing to pay and a seller is willing to accept.

Tangible Assets

Valuing tangible assets is a more straightforward exercise than valuing intangible assets such as goodwill. The price of dental equipment is listed in catalogs, and contractors can estimate buildout and remodel costs. Locating similar office space is problematic but not impossible. A seller places a high value on equipment and fixtures when they are in situ, otherwise used dental equipment carries little resale value. A seller has already depreciated tangible assets and reaped the tax shelter and the book value (accounting and tax residual value) of the equipment and furniture, and the leasehold is zero. Dental equipment does have an operational life beyond its depreciated life, but the resale market for used dental equipment is so thin that it might as well be nonexistent. In short, outside of the dental equipment being in operational order and in place, it has very low to zero market value, and the same holds for leasehold improvements, fixtures, and furniture, which are depreciated to a zero book value. In the end, just as with goodwill, the value of tangible assets is higher in the eyes of the seller than a buyer.

Outside of dental equipment being in operational order and in place, it has very low to zero market value, and the same holds for leasehold improvements, fixtures, and furniture.

Negotiation

In theory, to arrive at the final purchase price of an existing practice, the present value of the intangible asset goodwill is added to the tangible asset value. But, is this the correct price or a comfortable price? From day 1, can the practice's operational expense, loan payment, and personal expense be maintained solely by practice revenue? If so, is there an upside to growth? Is the value of an existing staff in terms of institutional memory, salary, and work ethic compatible with your vision and mission? Is the existing staff a positive or negative asset? Are you willing to walk away from the deal?

When you decide to purchase an existing dental practice, it is often convenient to enlist the help of a practice broker and an attorney to locate a desirable practice, determine its value, negotiate the terms, and execute a contract. There are four immutable facts to remember about the valuation of a dental practice:

1. Valuation is an art. There is no expert, spot-on formula.
2. Garbage in, garbage out. The quality of the data is paramount.
3. Uncertainty is the only certainty. There is no guarantee.
4. The ultimate value of a practice is the price a purchaser is willing to pay and the seller is willing to accept.

Debt Leverage and the Practice Loan

Whether you purchase an existing practice or start a new practice, a loan from a financial institution is required and prudent because funding a practice entirely from personal cash resources may be risky. A dental practice loan is the first in a series of loan transactions that occur throughout a career, and a large part of your financial strategy will be to positively leverage borrowing power (ie, debt) to increase your future revenue, income, and assets. Purchasing a Porsche is an example of negative leverage, ie, borrowed money invested in an asset that quickly loses value without producing cash flow. The utility between a Porsche and a Prius is equal. The control and leverage exercised through the judicious use of loan funds and the terms of the loan set the tone for the financial growth of the dental enterprise.

negative leverage
Borrowed money invested in an asset that quickly loses value without producing cash flow.

The control and leverage exercised through the judicious use of loan funds and the terms of the loan set the tone for the financial growth of the dental enterprise.

A practice loan is a package for equipment, supplies, leasehold improvement, buildouts, furnishings, and fixtures, while additional funds are requested for the practice's intangible goodwill. Real estate, such as a professional condominium, is sometimes rolled in, and the term (length) of the loan extended.

The essential items to know about a loan are the principal amount; the loan rate, which is expressed as the annual percentage rate (APR); and the term of the loan, which is expressed in months. The term for a dental practice loan usually runs from 36 to 120 months.

Loan Rate

The loan rate is tied to a benchmark like the prime rate or the recently introduced and presumably more stable London Interbank Offered Rate (LIBOR). Both the prime rate and LIBOR are published in the newspaper's financial section. To this loan rate are appended other costs like application, processing, and credit report fees; points; and other charges that effectively raise the total lending rate. Together the loan rate, fees, and charges are added together to arrive at the effective APR, which allows a potential borrower to compare apples to apples when shopping for loans. The APR can be fixed, variable, or mixed for the term of the loan.

Additional Loan Requirements

Lenders might impose additional loan requirements, such as a down payment of as much as 10%, which is required for a small business administration (SBA)–guaranteed loan. A cosigner who has assets to attach to the loan in case of default is sometimes required, and prepayment penalties for early payoff may apply. A term life insurance policy in the amount of the loan with the lender named as the beneficiary may be required as either a separate transaction or an addition to the loan amount (see chapter 5).

Calculating Payments

amortization ***(def 2)***
Gradual repayment of a loan in installments that are applied to both interest and principal.

An amortization table takes the principal amount, the APR, and the terms of the loan and computes the fixed total monthly payment, the pro rata monthly interest, and the principal throughout the term of the loan. As the loan matures, the interest portion of the monthly payment becomes smaller and the principal portion gets larger. Sometimes a much lower monthly payment is made that does not fully amortize the loan over its

Table 7-3 Amortization table for a hypothetical dental practice loan

Principal borrowed:	$500,000
Total payments:	120
Annual interest rate:	6%
Monthly payment:	$5,551
Total interest paid:	$166,122

Payment	Principal ($)	Interest ($)	Cumulative principal ($)	Cumulative interest ($)	Principal balance ($)
1	3,051.03	2,500.00	3,051.03	2,500.00	496,948.97
2	3,066.29	2,484.74	6,117.32	4,984.74	493,882.68
3	3,081.62	2,469.41	9,198.94	7,454.15	490,801.06
4	3,097.02	2,454.01	12,295.96	9,908.16	487,704.04
5	3,112.51	2,438.52	15,408.47	12,346.68	484,591.53
6	3,128.07	2,422.96	18,536.54	14,769.64	481,463.46
7	3,143.71	2,407.32	21,680.25	17,176.96	478,319.75
8	3,159.43	2,391.60	24,839.68	19,568.56	475,160.32
9	3,175.23	2,375.80	28,014.91	21,944.36	471,985.09
10	3,191.10	2,359.93	31,206.01	24,304.29	468,793.99
11	3,207.06	2,343.97	34,413.07	26,648.26	465,586.93
12	3,223.10	2,327.93	37,636.17	28,976.19	462,363.83
↓	↓	↓	↓	↓	↓
118	5,468.59	82.44	488,981.44	166,040.10	11,018.56
119	5,495.94	55.09	494,477.38	166,095.19	5,522.62
120	5,523.42	27.61	500,000.00	166,122.80	0.00

entire term, leaving one final large balloon payment to be paid at the end of the term.

A hypothetical dental practice loan for $500,000 amortized for 10 years, or 120 months, at a 6% APR has a fixed monthly payment of $5,551, or $66,622 annually (Table 7-3). If this were a loan you were applying for, you would have to ask yourself if the free cash flow of the practice could cover this monthly payment or if you need to seek different terms. Use

an online loan amortization calculator to change the principal, term, and APR to give you an idea of the sensitivity of the payment amount to each variable. Loan amortization calculators can automatically calculate monthly loan payments and generate amortization tables with the pro rata monthly interest and principal amounts.

Working Capital

working capital
A preapproved pool of money that is tapped by the borrower as needed for unexpected expenses or cash shortages.

line of credit
A revolving cash account accessed by writing a check on the account.

Working capital is a preapproved pool of money that is tapped by the borrower as needed for unexpected expenses or cash shortages. Working capital is often obtained through a line of credit that is a distinct and separate account from the practice loan. A line of credit is a revolving cash account accessed by writing a check on the account. Interest accrues only on the amount of money used and not on the entire line of credit itself. The APR on a line of credit is substantially higher than that on a fixed rate loan; in fact, interest rates can be so high on a line of credit that it should be used sparingly and only in short-term emergency situations. As money accessed from a line of credit is repaid, it is immediately available to borrow again (ie, the credit line revolves). A line of credit is a good way to pay bills in those times of unexpected cash flow shortages that often occur in a startup dental practice.

Dental practice loans can be obtained for up to $500,000 with no down payment and no cosigners. The debt is recorded with the state. Late payment or default can result in a lower credit score and liens placed against the property. A loan payment negatively affects cash flow for many years, even as the tax shelter aspect of depreciation declines. This means the payment is made even if the asset is no longer deducted on the income tax return to shelter income. Be wise. Be judicious. Buy only what you need, what you will use, and what you can afford.

Buy only what you need, what you will use, and what you can afford.

Applying for the Loan

Plan to apply for your dental practice loan at least 9 months before opening the door, and at least 1 year prior to opening the door if the practice

LOAN AMORTIZATION CALCULATORS

- www.bretwhissel.net/cgi-bin/amortize
- www.bankrate.com/calculators/mortgages/loan-calculator.aspx
- www.amortization-calc.com/

requires extensive buildout and leasehold improvement. Expect to spend a month assembling documentation and another month obtaining funding. Health care–oriented lenders approve loans based solely on a dental degree, so most don't require collateral, cosigners, or a down payment. In the 2009 economic recession, dental practice loan funds were scarce and dear but still available from banks and finance companies. Some lenders fund and service their own loans, while others process the application and pass it on to the SBA to fund. Ask questions of every lender. Look for competitive terms on the APR, down payment, and collateral, and review the lender's track record.

Plan to apply for your dental practice loan at least 9 months before opening the door, and at least 1 year prior to opening the door if the practice requires extensive buildout and leasehold improvement.

The application process requires you to provide a basic information form, loan amount, use of funds, office lease agreement, personal bank account statement(s), income tax return(s), and a business plan with a meticulous monthly pro forma cash flow projected over 2 years (see chapter 10 and appendix II). A business plan usually includes a definite location, lease, floor plan, estimated buildout and remodel, equipment, supplies, furnishings, and fixtures.

A thorough accounting of personal debts and expenses is essential. A major source of personal debt is your student loan. Consolidate any student loans you have into a single loan to improve your cash flow, financial profile, and credit score.

Consolidate any student loans you have into a single loan to improve your cash flow, financial profile, and credit score.

If this is a practice purchase loan, include the purchase agreement, the seller's bank account record(s), seller's income tax return(s), office lease, and any other seller documentation requested by the lender. Be prepared to supply all documents in a timely fashion. Requesting the required documents from the seller before applying to the lender will keep you from wasting your time with needless back-and-forth correspondence. Append all documents to the application.

Pro forma cash flow

The most important element in a practice loan application is the pro forma cash flow. Although approval for a dental practice loan is based in large part on your dental degree and credit score, as well as the lender's judgment of your character and potential for future high income, cash flow estimates from an existing practice or pro forma cash flow are weighted the most heavily. The pro forma should include personal cash needs and sources of additional income like associate wage and spousal wage. Cash needs ebb and flow throughout the year and don't follow averages. Including personal cash needs provides a realistic assessment of how much cash is really required on a month-to-month basis. A realistic

pro forma
Forecasted or informal; based on assumptions and hypothetical information.

A realistic pro forma cash flow gives the lender a thorough analysis that shows that you won't be short at the end of the month and unable to pay current liabilities, including the practice loan.

pro forma cash flow gives the lender a thorough analysis that shows that you won't be short at the end of the month and unable to pay current liabilities, including the practice loan.

Examples of specific lenders' terms

Bank of America

In 2009, Bank of America Practice Solutions was offering 100% financing for new startup practices for equipment, cabinetry, office furniture, fixtures, and supplies; renovation and construction; architecture, design, and management consultant fees; and working capital. It had fixed rate terms for up to 15 years with deferred, graduated, and interest-only payments for up to 6 months. The rate was locked for up to 12 months to give the dentist time to start the practice with a guaranteed loan and rate.[1]

Excel National Bank

In 2009, Excel National Bank was offering SBA loans for up to $2,000,000 with a 90% loan-to-value, and they were also offering 3-, 5-, and 10-year repayment terms without a prepayment penalty.[2]

Matsco

Matsco (a Wells Fargo company) provides practice acquisition and startup financing for dentists. In 2009, they were offering up to 100% financing, fixed rate loans, deferred payment for practice acquisitions, and graduated payment programs for practice startups. Working capital lines of credit were also available.[3]

Credit Score and Report

Financial institutions use a credit score derived from credit reports to judge your creditworthiness and ability to repay the loan. It's the single most important factor in getting a loan at a competitive rate. Even a penurious dental student with only a few assets has already amassed a detailed credit history.

Fair Isaac Corporation (FICO) credit score
A three-digit number based on credit reports that is used to gauge your credit worthiness.

Fair Isaac Corporation (FICO) Credit Score

The Fair Isaac Corporation (FICO) credit score is a three-digit number used to gauge your creditworthiness. It is calculated based on Equifax and

TransUnion credit reports; as of 2009, a FICO credit score based on an Experian credit report is no longer available.

Credit scores range from 300 to 850, with a score of 800–850 being outstanding, 750–799 being excellent, 700–749 being good, and 650–699 being fair. A score below 650 makes it difficult to obtain any loan at all. The average FICO score is 690. With the 2009 financial meltdown, lenders focus much more on credit risk and creditworthiness and look for FICO scores above 760.[4]

The FICO score is weighed on a number of factors:

- 35% reflects payment history–Are bills paid on time?
- 30% reflects amounts currently owed–How much of a balance is carried on a credit limit?
- 15% reflects the length of credit history–The longer the credit history, the better.
- 10% reflects new credit–How many accounts have you recently opened?
- 10% reflects the types of credit used–Is there a mix of accounts: loan, credit card, mortgage?

The terms of any loan become more favorable as your FICO score rises; in fact, your FICO credit score and credit history are the most significant factors in the assessment of your loan application.

The terms of any loan become more favorable as your FICO score rises; in fact, your FICO credit score and credit history are the most significant factors in the assessment of your loan application.

Factors that negatively affect your credit score

Major factors that negatively impact a FICO score are late payments, collection accounts, judgments, general liens, tax liens, pursuing too many credit cards, using credit limits to their maximum limit, and bankruptcy. If a credit account is sent to a collection agency and is subsequently paid in full, the collection account remains on the report and negatively impacts the credit score for 7 years. Closing the account doesn't make it go away.

Credit reports and credit scores don't give a free pass to a penurious student who overextends his or her credit and pays bills late. A negative but accurate report can't be improved instantly, and there is no immediate recourse to mitigate or erase an accurate entry. Only time will eliminate the ding from your record. Be prudent, be diligent, and actively manage your credit score.

Credit reports and credit scores don't give a free pass to a penurious student who overextends his or her credit and pays bills late.

Raising your credit score

Although a negative score cannot be improved instantly, you can still raise your credit score by making sure to pay all of your bills on time. If

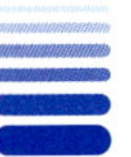

you miss a payment, get current and stay current because the 2009 version of the FICO score is very sensitive to payment history.[5] Keep balances low on credit cards and other revolving credit lines such as department store charge cards, and open as few new credit accounts as possible. In addition, don't shop for more than one type of loan (eg, practice, car, or home) in a short period of time so it doesn't appear that you're seeking multiple loans.

Reviewing your credit score and credit reports

FICO charges a fee to see your credit score on its website, but a free credit report from each credit report bureau is available once a year from a Federal Trade Commission–approved central website. Request a copy of your credit reports at least once a year to monitor them for accuracy, and alert each bureau with any discrepancies and unrecorded closed accounts.

Financial Statements

The balance sheet, income statement, and cash flow statement are financial statements prepared using the principles of GAAP. Publicly traded companies use financial statements and GAAP to provide uniform and transparent financial information to shareholders in the marketplace. However, a sole proprietor never needs to use double-entry bookkeeping and accrual accounting or prepare financial reports that meet GAAP standards, but he or she does need to prepare some financial statements to build a business strategy and maintain financial control.

Balance Sheet

As described in chapter 1, the balance sheet is a statement of financial position that describes assets and liabilities at a given date to calculate net worth (Fig 7-1).

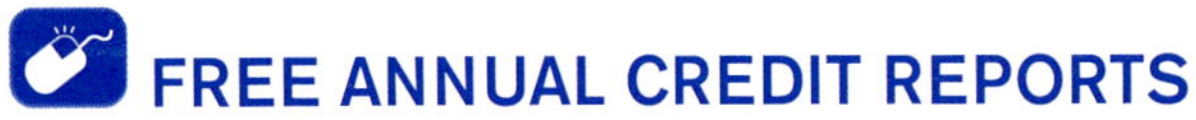
FREE ANNUAL CREDIT REPORTS

- www.annualcreditreport.com

Balance Sheet

	Assets	
Current assets		
	Checking account	$5,000
	Savings account	$5,000
	Brokerage account	$10,000
Noncurrent assets		
	Porsche	$95,000
	Jewelry	$50,000
Intangible assets		
	Dental degree	$150,000
Total assets		$315,000
	Liabilities	
Current liabilities		
	Credit card debt	$2,000
	Porsche loan—current portion	$25,000
	Student loan—current portion	$15,000
Long-term liabilities		
	Porsche loan	$70,000
	Student loan	$135,000
Total liabilities		$247,000
	Equity	
Net worth		$68,000

Fig 7-1 Sample balance sheet. Note that the dental degree is included as an intangible asset.

Assets

Assets can be current or noncurrent. A current asset can be converted to cash in a short period of time (eg, accounts receivable), as opposed to a noncurrent asset, which has a life span of more than a year and is difficult to turn into cash. Dental equipment is an example of a noncurrent tangible asset, and goodwill is an example of noncurrent intangible asset.

current asset
Asset that can be converted to cash in a short period of time (eg, accounts receivable).

noncurrent asset
An asset with a life span of more than a year that is difficult to turn into cash (eg, dental equipment or practice goodwill).

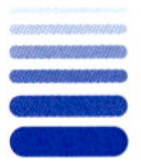

Liabilities

current liabilities
Debts to be repaid within a year.

long-term liabilities
Debts to be repaid over a period longer than a year.

Liabilities can be current or long term. Current liabilities, such as a laboratory bill, are due within a year. The portion of a Porsche car loan due this calendar year is a current liability. Alternatively, long-term liabilities are debts to be repaid over a period longer than a year, so the portion of a Porsche car loan due beyond a year is a long-term liability.

Owner's equity

Owner's equity for a sole proprietor is the same as net worth. In an unincorporated sole proprietorship, all profits are deemed distributed at the end of the year; therefore, they are taxed for that year. There is no retained earnings line in a sole proprietorship.

Ratios

The balance sheet is useful for visualizing important ratios such as debt to current assets and debt to equity. These ratios give a sense of the debt leverage and the ability to pay debt obligations through current assets. In this way, the balance sheet gives a sense of liquidity and whether the value of the assets significantly outweighs liabilities; otherwise, bankruptcy may loom. It can also give the owner a snapshot of net worth, ie, how much wealth has been accumulated.

Income Statement and Cash Flow Statement

accrual basis accounting
Method of accounting that recognizes revenue when the service is rendered and expense when it is incurred.

cash basis accounting
Method of accounting universally used by dentists that recognizes revenue when collected and expense when paid.

The income statement, also called the *profit and loss statement, earnings statement,* or *operating statement,* reflects practice operation over a specific period of time, usually a calendar year. It records revenue and the related expenses used to generate that income, including the noncash, tax-related expenses depreciation and amortization. Income statements are useful for business entities that are obligated to meet GAAP standards, which require accrual basis accounting, in which revenue is recognized when the service is rendered and expense recognized when it is incurred. Dentists, however, universally use cash basis accounting, where revenue is recognized when collected and expense when paid.

For our purposes, the cash flow statement is the most useful report. Unlike the income statement, it only recognizes cash events, ignoring depreciation and amortization since these are noncash items. However, for most dentists, the office checkbook (described later in this chapter) is a proxy for a cash flow statement.

Depreciation, Amortization, and Expensing

As explained earlier in this chapter, depreciation refers to the conversion of the cost of a long-lived tangible asset, such as a piece of dental equipment, into an expense over a period of years, while amortization refers to the conversion of the cost of an intangible asset, such as goodwill, into an expense over a period of years. On the other hand, expensing occurs when you fully convert the cost of a long-lived tangible asset into an expense during the year it was purchased. The 2009 Internal Revenue Service (IRS) Section 179 allows for immediate deduction (expensing versus depreciation) of up to $250,000 in long-lived dental purchases.

expensing
Fully converting the cost of a long-lived tangible asset into an expense during the year it was purchased.

Depreciation

Depreciation can be calculated in several ways, including straight-line depreciation or accelerated methods such as double declining balance and sum of the years' digits. In straight-line depreciation, the cost of the asset is divided by its expected life. For example, a $10,500 dental chair with an expected useful life of 7 years and no salvage value is depreciated at the annual rate of $1,500 per year. This means that you could deduct $1,500 on the income statement and Schedule C each year for 7 years to reduce income and thereby reduce your income tax, even though after the first year it is a noncash event.

straight-line depreciation
The cost of the asset is divided by its expected life in years.

Accelerated depreciation allows for a faster tax deduction, which reduces current income taxes and results in a higher tax shield. Of course, expensing equipment is the ultimate opportunity to use accelerated depreciation. Consult an accountant to determine the appropriate tax strategy and depreciation method for you.

accelerated depreciation
Methods such as double declining balance and sum of the years' digits that allow for a faster tax deduction, which reduces current income taxes and results in a higher tax shield.

Amortization

Amortization has two meanings–both have been used in this chapter–that are often confused, misunderstood, and misapplied. In this section, it is used to mean the conversion of the cost of an intangible asset into an expense over a period of years. Amortization is entered onto financial statements such as the income statement. In another context, amortization has a completely different definition that refers to a regular cash payment made to pay down a debt (ie, amortize a debt) that is calculated using an amortization table. Goodwill is an example of an intangible asset that is amortized. Like depreciation, it is a noncash, bookkeeping, tax-related entry.

Federal Reporting

Depreciation and amortization are reported on Form 4562 and then transferred to Schedule C. Expensed equipment under Section 179 is likewise calculated on Form 4562, then carried over to Schedule C. Only small dental instruments (eg, hand instruments) are deducted directly on Schedule C.

Checkbook

Your most useful financial tool as a dentist is your office checkbook. It represents cash basis accounting because it records only actual cash revenue and expense transactions. Revenue is the cash, check, or credit card deposit actually made. You can buy a real cup of coffee with real money from cash basis accounting revenue. Expense is what is actually paid out by cash or check. An expense paid with a credit card isn't counted until the credit card statement is actually paid.

Although you may visit the balance sheet on occasion to see how much you're worth, you live daily in the checkbook.

Accounts receivable and accounts payable are recorded elsewhere, not in the checkbook. The checkbook is a proxy for a cash flow statement. Although you may visit the balance sheet on occasion to see how much you're worth, you live daily in the checkbook.

Checkbook Management Software

To manage your checkbook account, select a software program that works for you. The day of the no. 2 lead pencil and green accounting sheet is long past. An example of an accessible, efficient, user-friendly program is Quicken from Intuit, which is available in PC or Mac format. The program records and organizes income and expense, then automatically assembles customized reports. It can reconcile the checkbook, matching every dollar collected with a deposit, every charge with an invoice, and every payment with a cancelled check to arrive at an ending balance that mirrors the bank statement, giving you a balanced checkbook.

Sample Chart of Accounts

Revenue	
Patient check	
Credit card	
Insurance check	
	100.0
Expenses	% of revenue
Wages	
Salary—Staff	16.1
Salary—Hygienist	10.0
Payroll tax	5.3
Staff benefit	1.2
Dental	
Laboratory	7.2
Dental supply	6.0
Rent	4.9
Office	
Stationery and supplies	2.6
Insurance	1.8
Legal and accounting	1.7
Computer and software	1.5
Advertising and marketing	1.2
Business tax	1.0
Telephone	1.0
Utilities	1.0
Repair and maintenance	0.8
Dues and subscriptions	0.5
Continuing education	0.3
Laundry	0.3
Janitorial	0.2
Miscellaneous	2.0
Total operational expense	66.6

Fig 7-2 Sample chart of accounts.

Chart of accounts

A checkbook software program will include a chart of accounts, which establishes categories of revenue and expense (Fig 7-2). The first step in developing a chart of accounts is to define and name categories that are uniquely meaningful to your practice. There is no standard, official, or best chart of accounts. A new practice might separate revenue by patient check, credit card, and insurance check, and wages might be separated into front office, back office, and hygiene expense. Loan payments might be listed separately.

Your software program will use this chart of accounts to generate reports that will assist you in making management decisions and preparing income tax returns. Reports generated based on these accounts give managers the ability to gauge the effect of wages, overtime, benefits, laboratory fees, and dental supplies against revenue. There are also dental industry benchmark ratios that compare certain expense categories against revenue, thereby allowing a dentist to gauge whether his or her practice is in line with similar practices.

Income Tax

wage
Money earned from employment.

revenue
Money collected in the practice.

income
What is left to the dentist after deducting expenses from revenue.

A federal income tax return must be filed annually by April 15th for the preceding calendar year. When filing an income tax return, it is important to understand the differences between wage, income, and revenue. Wage is money earned from employment; revenue is money collected in the practice; and income is what is left to the dentist after deducting paid expenses from revenue.

For the sake of simplicity, let's presume that you are an unincorporated sole proprietor reporting on a cash basis. There are two accounts not recorded for cash reporting and income tax purposes–accounts receivable and accounts payable. As discussed previously, accounts receivable is money owed to you but not collected, eg, an insurance check payment that is still being processed. Accounts payable is money owed by you but not paid, as in the case of a laboratory fabricated crown that has been cemented, but the monthly laboratory bill has not yet been paid out of the checkbook. The single accounting event that doesn't follow the cash accounting convention is the wages paid to employees. Since the Social Security Administration and the IRS share information, a dentist must report all wages paid in the calendar year to the IRS, including the last payroll check issued in December, even if that employee's wage check doesn't clear the bank until the following calendar year.

accounts payable
Money owed but not paid.

The single accounting event that doesn't follow the cash accounting convention is wages paid to employees, which must be reported when the checks are issued, regardless of whether they have cleared the bank.

Box 7-3 Common tax schedules and forms reported on Form 1040

Schedule A–Itemized Deductions
Schedule B–Interest and Ordinary Dividends
Schedule C–Profit or Loss from Business (Sole Proprietorship)
Schedule D–Capital Gains and Losses
Schedule SE–Self Employment Tax
Form 4562–Depreciation and Amortization
Form 8889–Health Savings Account (HSA)
Form W-2–Wage & Tax Statement

Form 1040

The US Individual Income Tax Return Form 1040 is a summary of income, adjustments to income, deductions, and credits that is filed annually. Most amounts are bottom-line figures transferred from other schedules and forms (Box 7-3).

Page 1: Adjusted gross income

Page 1 is where earned wage from employment (Form W-2), Schedule C income (or loss) from the dental practice, and deductions for items such as a health savings account (HSA), self-employed health insurance, and an individual retirement account (IRA) are entered to arrive at the adjusted gross income (Fig 7-3).

Form W-2

Income earned as an employee (ie, wage) is reported on Form W-2. Your employer reports the amount of state and federal income taxes withheld, including Social Security and Medicare. One-half of the taxes for Social Security and Medicare is paid through an employee's wage, while the other half is paid by the employer on the employee's behalf as an employment tax. Employers must distribute a W-2 to each employee in a timely manner immediately following the end of the calendar year.

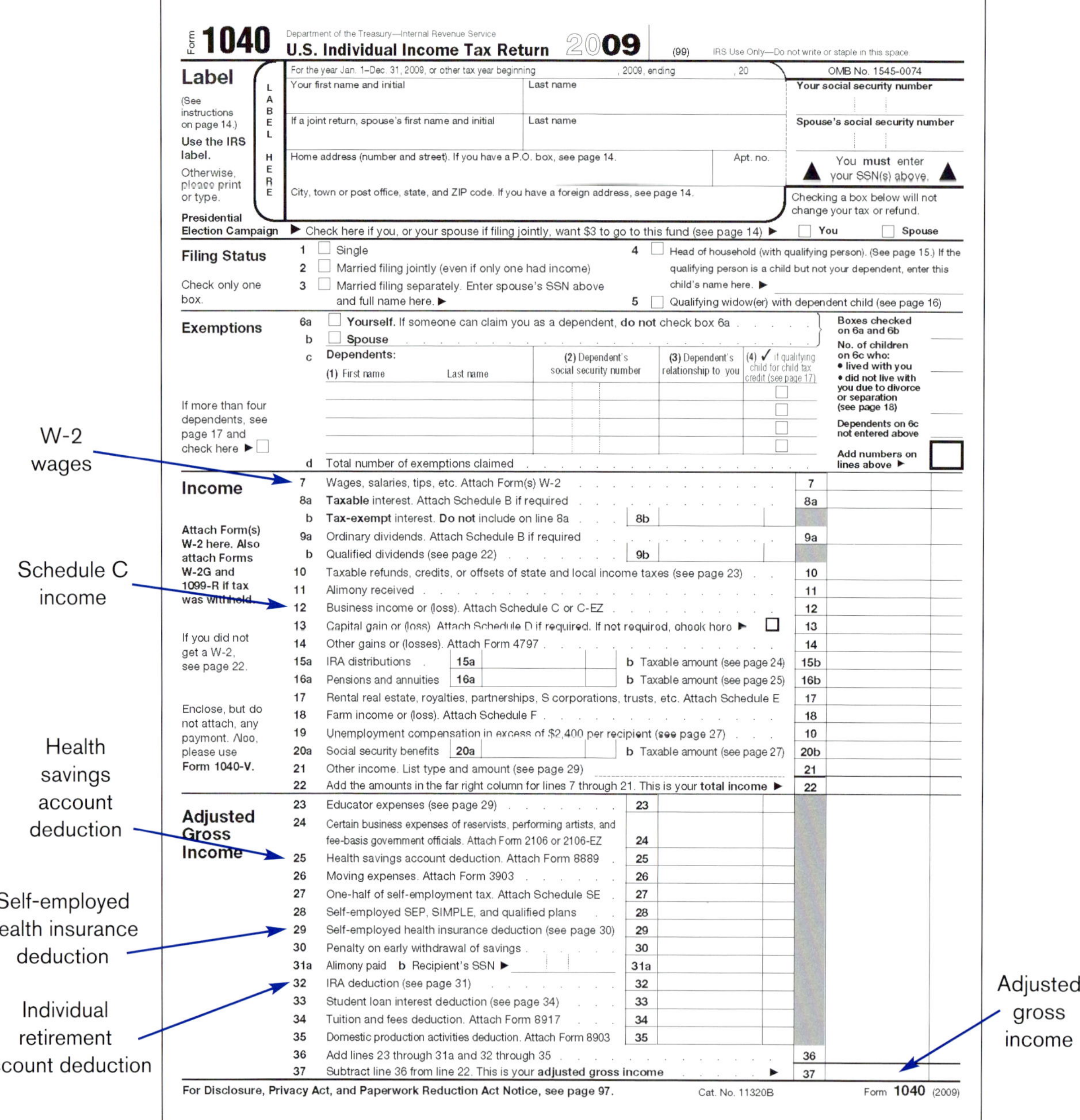

Form **1040** Department of the Treasury—Internal Revenue Service
U.S. Individual Income Tax Return 2009 (99) IRS Use Only—Do not write or staple in this space.

For the year Jan. 1–Dec. 31, 2009, or other tax year beginning , 2009, ending , 20 OMB No. 1545-0074

Label (See instructions on page 14.) Use the IRS label. Otherwise, please print or type. LABEL HERE

Your first name and initial | Last name | **Your social security number**

If a joint return, spouse's first name and initial | Last name | **Spouse's social security number**

Home address (number and street). If you have a P.O. box, see page 14. | Apt. no. | ▲ You **must** enter your SSN(s) above. ▲

City, town or post office, state, and ZIP code. If you have a foreign address, see page 14. | Checking a box below will not change your tax or refund.

Presidential Election Campaign ▶ Check here if you, or your spouse if filing jointly, want $3 to go to this fund (see page 14) ▶ ☐ You ☐ Spouse

Filing Status
Check only one box.
1 ☐ Single
2 ☐ Married filing jointly (even if only one had income)
3 ☐ Married filing separately. Enter spouse's SSN above and full name here. ▶
4 ☐ Head of household (with qualifying person). (See page 15.) If the qualifying person is a child but not your dependent, enter this child's name here. ▶
5 ☐ Qualifying widow(er) with dependent child (see page 16)

Exemptions
6a ☐ **Yourself.** If someone can claim you as a dependent, **do not** check box 6a
b ☐ **Spouse**
c **Dependents:** (1) First name Last name | (2) Dependent's social security number | (3) Dependent's relationship to you | (4) ✓ if qualifying child for child tax credit (see page 17)
If more than four dependents, see page 17 and check here ▶ ☐
d Total number of exemptions claimed
Boxes checked on 6a and 6b
No. of children on 6c who: • lived with you • did not live with you due to divorce or separation (see page 18)
Dependents on 6c not entered above
Add numbers on lines above ▶

Income
Attach Form(s) W-2 here. Also attach Forms W-2G and 1099-R if tax was withheld.
If you did not get a W-2, see page 22.
Enclose, but do not attach, any payment. Also, please use **Form 1040-V.**

7 Wages, salaries, tips, etc. Attach Form(s) W-2 — 7
8a **Taxable** interest. Attach Schedule B if required — 8a
b **Tax-exempt** interest. **Do not** include on line 8a — 8b
9a Ordinary dividends. Attach Schedule B if required — 9a
b Qualified dividends (see page 22) — 9b
10 Taxable refunds, credits, or offsets of state and local income taxes (see page 23) — 10
11 Alimony received — 11
12 Business income or (loss). Attach Schedule C or C-EZ — 12
13 Capital gain or (loss). Attach Schedule D if required. If not required, check here ▶ ☐ — 13
14 Other gains or (losses). Attach Form 4797 — 14
15a IRA distributions 15a | b Taxable amount (see page 24) — 15b
16a Pensions and annuities 16a | b Taxable amount (see page 25) — 16b
17 Rental real estate, royalties, partnerships, S corporations, trusts, etc. Attach Schedule E — 17
18 Farm income or (loss). Attach Schedule F — 18
19 Unemployment compensation in excess of $2,400 per recipient (see page 27) — 19
20a Social security benefits 20a | b Taxable amount (see page 27) — 20b
21 Other income. List type and amount (see page 29) — 21
22 Add the amounts in the far right column for lines 7 through 21. This is your **total income** ▶ — 22

Adjusted Gross Income
23 Educator expenses (see page 29) — 23
24 Certain business expenses of reservists, performing artists, and fee-basis government officials. Attach Form 2106 or 2106-EZ — 24
25 Health savings account deduction. Attach Form 8889 — 25
26 Moving expenses. Attach Form 3903 — 26
27 One-half of self-employment tax. Attach Schedule SE — 27
28 Self-employed SEP, SIMPLE, and qualified plans — 28
29 Self-employed health insurance deduction (see page 30) — 29
30 Penalty on early withdrawal of savings — 30
31a Alimony paid b Recipient's SSN ▶ — 31a
32 IRA deduction (see page 31) — 32
33 Student loan interest deduction (see page 34) — 33
34 Tuition and fees deduction. Attach Form 8917 — 34
35 Domestic production activities deduction. Attach Form 8903 — 35
36 Add lines 23 through 31a and 32 through 35 — 36
37 Subtract line 36 from line 22. This is your **adjusted gross income** ▶ — 37

For Disclosure, Privacy Act, and Paperwork Reduction Act Notice, see page 97. Cat. No. 11320B Form **1040** (2009)

Fig 7-3 Sample Form 1040, page 1.

Schedule C

Schedule C–Profit or Loss from Business (Sole Proprietorship) is where the dental business summarizes its revenue and expense by category (Fig 7-4). The noncash account for depreciation, expensing, and amortization of equipment, furnishings, fixtures, and leasehold improvements from

SCHEDULE C (Form 1040)

Department of the Treasury
Internal Revenue Service (99)

Profit or Loss From Business
(Sole Proprietorship)

▶ Partnerships, joint ventures, etc., generally must file Form 1065 or 1065-B.
▶ Attach to Form 1040, 1040NR, or 1041. ▶ See Instructions for Schedule C (Form 1040).

OMB No. 1545-0074
2009
Attachment Sequence No. **09**

Name of proprietor | **Social security number (SSN)**

A Principal business or profession, including product or service (see page C-2 of the instructions) | **B Enter code from pages C-9, 10, & 11** ▶

C Business name. If no separate business name, leave blank. | **D Employer ID number (EIN), if any**

E Business address (including suite or room no.) ▶
City, town or post office, state, and ZIP code

F Accounting method: **(1)** ☐ Cash **(2)** ☐ Accrual **(3)** ☐ Other (specify) ▶

G Did you "materially participate" in the operation of this business during 2009? If "No," see page C-3 for limit on losses ☐ **Yes** ☐ **No**

H If you started or acquired this business during 2009, check here . . . ▶ ☐

Part I Income

1	Gross receipts or sales. **Caution.** See page C-4 and check the box if: • This income was reported to you on Form W-2 and the "Statutory employee" box on that form was checked, or • You are a member of a qualified joint venture reporting only rental real estate income not subject to self-employment tax. Also see page C-3 for limit on losses. ▶ ☐	1	
2	Returns and allowances	2	
3	Subtract line 2 from line 1	3	
4	Cost of goods sold (from line 42 on page 2)	4	
5	**Gross profit.** Subtract line 4 from line 3	5	
6	Other income, including federal and state gasoline or fuel tax credit or refund (see page C-4)	6	
7	**Gross income.** Add lines 5 and 6 ▶	7	

Part II Expenses. Enter expenses for business use of your home **only** on line 30.

8	Advertising	8		18	Office expense	18	
9	Car and truck expenses (see page C-4)	9		19	Pension and profit-sharing plans	19	
				20	Rent or lease (see page C-6):		
10	Commissions and fees	10		a	Vehicles, machinery, and equipment	20a	
11	Contract labor (see page C-4)	11		b	Other business property	20b	
12	Depletion	12		21	Repairs and maintenance	21	
13	Depreciation and section 179 expense deduction (not included in Part III) (see page C-5)	13		22	Supplies (not included in Part III)	22	
				23	Taxes and licenses	23	
				24	Travel, meals, and entertainment:		
				a	Travel	24a	
14	Employee benefit programs (other than on line 19)	14		b	Deductible meals and entertainment (see page C-6)	24b	
15	Insurance (other than health)	15		25	Utilities	25	
16	Interest:			26	Wages (less employment credits)	26	
a	Mortgage (paid to banks, etc.)	16a		27	Other expenses (from line 48 on page 2)	27	
b	Other	16b					
17	Legal and professional services	17					

28	**Total expenses** before expenses for business use of home. Add lines 8 through 27 ▶	28	
29	Tentative profit or (loss). Subtract line 28 from line 7	29	
30	Expenses for business use of your home. Attach **Form 8829**	30	
31	**Net profit or (loss).** Subtract line 30 from line 29. • If a profit, enter on both **Form 1040, line 12,** and **Schedule SE, line 2,** or on **Form 1040NR, line 13** (if you checked the box on line 1, see page C-7). Estates and trusts, enter on **Form 1041, line 3.** • If a loss, you **must** go to line 32.	31	
32	If you have a loss, check the box that describes your investment in this activity (see page C-7). • If you checked 32a, enter the loss on both **Form 1040, line 12,** and **Schedule SE, line 2,** or on **Form 1040NR, line 13** (if you checked the box on line 1, see the line 31 instructions on page C-7). Estates and trusts, enter on **Form 1041, line 3.** • If you checked 32b, you **must** attach **Form 6198.** Your loss may be limited.	32a ☐ All investment is at risk. 32b ☐ Some investment is not at risk.	

For Paperwork Reduction Act Notice, see page C-9 of the instructions. Cat. No. 11334P **Schedule C (Form 1040) 2009**

Revenue actually collected

Itemized expenses from separate sheet

Net profit transferred to Form 1040 page 1

Fig 7-4 Sample Schedule C—Profit or Loss from Business (Sole Proprietorship).

Form 4562 is entered on Schedule C. Each individual sole proprietor business requires a separate Schedule C, whether it is a private practice, independent contractor business, or any other separate businesses (eg, authoring a book). Remember that wage from employment as an associate dentist or professor at a university is not entered on Schedule C; rather, it is entered separately on page 1 of Form 1040.

Forms 1040 with an attached Schedule C have higher-than-average audit rates, so always keep detailed records to substantiate deductions.

Forms 1040 with an attached Schedule C have higher-than-average audit rates, so always keep detailed records to substantiate deductions. Certain business deductions that appear intuitively reasonable are often disallowed, and just because you have taken a deduction once or over many years without an audit doesn't automatically make them a qualified IRS business deduction. If you are subject to an income tax audit and have taken disallowed business deductions, you could be responsible for a payment of back taxes, interest, and penalties. If you're unsure whether an expense qualifies as a tax deduction, consult with a qualified accountant or attorney to determine whether certain business deductions can be defended as a legitimate business expense. Following are explanations of some commonly misunderstood deductions.

Principal on a dental school loan is only tax deductible in the year the loan was taken out.

Student loan deductions The interest paid on a student loan is a tax-deductible event reported directly on page 1 of Form 1040 (see line 33 in Fig 7-3). It is, however, subject to income limitations, and the current maximum deductible amount is $2,500. Principal on a dental school loan, on the other hand, is not usually tax deductible other than in the year the loan was taken out (ie, it may be a legitimate deduction only during the dental school year in which the tuition expense was incurred). The payment of the principal on the loan in subsequent years is not a business expense to be deducted on Schedule C. Any educational cost to prepare for a new profession such as law school is not deductible as a business expense; however, it may qualify as a tuition expense, subject to income limitations.

An automobile loan or lease payment is generally not deductible on a Schedule C.

Automobile loan or lease payment deductions An automobile loan or lease payment is generally not deductible on a Schedule C. Interest paid on an automobile loan is reported as a personal deduction on Schedule A only if the automobile loan is paid with a home equity loan; otherwise, it's a nondeductible personal expense.

If you are an employee using a company-owned or leased car, note that the personal use of an employer-provided vehicle is a fringe benefit that is generally taxable unless specifically excluded by law. Employees must substantiate their business use through adequate documentation to qualify as an excludable working-condition fringe benefit.

Medical insurance premium deductions The medical insurance premium payment for an unincorporated sole proprietor dentist is reported directly on Form 1040 as a personal deduction and not reported on Schedule C. However, employee medical insurance premiums paid by the dentist are a dental business expense reported on Schedule C.

Uniform allowance deductions A uniform allowance expense for the dentist and staff is deducted on Schedule C if the uniform style isn't normally worn outside the office. For instance, a dress shirt, tie, and trousers that can be worn as personal apparel are not generally deductible as a business expense even if worn exclusively at the office. In other words, don't buy yourself an Armani suit expecting to be able to write it off. However, the cost of a blue cotton surgical scrub–as well as its associated laundry expense–is deductible.

A uniform allowance expense for the dentist and staff is deducted on Schedule C if the uniform style isn't normally worn outside the office.

Commuting expense deductions Commuting expenses between home and office such as gas, tolls, and garage fees are not considered practice expenses and are not usually tax deductible; however, the commute between separate dental offices on the same day may be deductible depending on the tax home. A tax home is a taxpayer's primary place of work regardless of his or her place of residence. If a taxpayer regularly works at two or more separate locations, his or her tax home is the general area of principal employment or business, as determined by such factors as the amount of time spent and income earned there. Expenses incurred by traveling to and from the minor place of employment are deductible expenses. This is the case, for instance, when a dentist practicing in San Francisco also teaches in Los Angeles or when a dentist is employed and earns wages in two different practices, with one practice located in New York City and the other in West Hartford, Connecticut. Transportation is deductible either on a cents per mile basis or based on actual expenses incurred by the commute between offices if you are going from one office to another in the same day, and possibly also for the commute to different offices on separate days depending on your tax home and your principal place of business. However, keep in mind that the expenditure for spending the night somewhere for business purposes is generally considered a *travel expense*, whereas the cost of getting from one place of business to another is a *transportation expense*.

tax home
A taxpayer's primary place of work regardless of his or her residence.

Page 2: Taxable income

Page 2 of Form 1040 (Fig 7-5) is where the standard deduction or itemized deductions from Schedule A are entered to arrive at taxable income. Self-employment tax (Schedule SE), any estimated quarterly income tax

Standard deduction or itemized deductions from Schedule A

Taxable income

Schedule SE—self-employment tax

Income tax

Total tax = income tax + self-employment tax

Estimated federal income tax quarterly payments

Bottom line tax liability due or refund owed

Form 1040 (2009) Page **2**

Tax and Credits

38 Amount from line 37 (adjusted gross income) . . . 38

39a Check if: { ☐ **You** were born before January 2, 1945, ☐ Blind. } Total boxes
☐ **Spouse** was born before January 2, 1945, ☐ Blind. } checked ▶ 39a

b If your spouse itemizes on a separate return or you were a dual-status alien, see page 35 and check here ▶ 39b☐

Standard Deduction for—
• People who check any box on line 39a, 39b, or 40b **or** who can be claimed as a dependent, see page 35.
• All others:
Single or Married filing separately, $5,700
Married filing jointly or Qualifying widow(er), $11,400
Head of household, $8,350

40a **Itemized deductions** (from Schedule A) **or** your **standard deduction** (see left margin) . . 40a

b If you are increasing your standard deduction by certain real estate taxes, new motor vehicle taxes, or a net disaster loss, attach Schedule L and check here (see page 35) . ▶ 40b☐

41 Subtract line 40a from line 38 . . . 41

42 **Exemptions.** If line 38 is $125,100 or less and you did not provide housing to a Midwestern displaced individual, multiply $3,650 by the number on line 6d. Otherwise, see page 37 . . 42

43 **Taxable income.** Subtract line 42 from line 41. If line 42 is more than line 41, enter -0- . . 43

44 **Tax** (see page 37). Check if any tax is from: a ☐ Form(s) 8814 b ☐ Form 4972 . 44

45 **Alternative minimum tax** (see page 40). Attach Form 6251 . . . 45

46 Add lines 44 and 45 . . . ▶ 46

47 Foreign tax credit. Attach Form 1116 if required . . . 47

48 Credit for child and dependent care expenses. Attach Form 2441 48

49 Education credits from Form 8863, line 29 . . . 49

50 Retirement savings contributions credit. Attach Form 8880 50

51 Child tax credit (see page 42) . . . 51

52 Credits from Form: a ☐ 8396 b ☐ 8839 c ☐ 5695 52

53 Other credits from Form: a ☐ 3800 b ☐ 8801 c ☐ 53

54 Add lines 47 through 53. These are your **total credits** . . . 54

55 Subtract line 54 from line 46. If line 54 is more than line 46, enter -0- . . . ▶ 55

Other Taxes

56 Self-employment tax. Attach Schedule SE . . . 56

57 Unreported social security and Medicare tax from Form: a ☐ 4137 b ☐ 8919 . . 57

58 Additional tax on IRAs, other qualified retirement plans, etc. Attach Form 5329 if required . . 58

59 Additional taxes: a ☐ AEIC payments b ☐ Household employment taxes. Attach Schedule H 59

60 Add lines 55 through 59. This is your **total tax** . . . ▶ 60

Payments

61 Federal income tax withheld from Forms W-2 and 1099 . . 61

62 2009 estimated tax payments and amount applied from 2008 return 62

If you have a qualifying child, attach Schedule EIC.

63 Making work pay and government retiree credits. Attach Schedule M 63

64a **Earned income credit (EIC)** . . . 64a

b Nontaxable combat pay election 64b

65 Additional child tax credit. Attach Form 8812 . . . 65

66 Refundable education credit from Form 8863, line 16 . . . 66

67 First-time homebuyer credit. Attach Form 5405 . . . 67

68 Amount paid with request for extension to file (see page 72) . 68

69 Excess social security and tier 1 RRTA tax withheld (see page 72) . 69

70 Credits from Form: a ☐ 2439 b ☐ 4136 c ☐ 8801 d ☐ 8885 70

71 Add lines 61, 62, 63, 64a, and 65 through 70. These are your **total payments** . . . ▶ 71

Refund

72 If line 71 is more than line 60, subtract line 60 from line 71. This is the amount you **overpaid** 72

Direct deposit? See page 73 and fill in 73b, 73c, and 73d, or Form 8888.

73a Amount of line 72 you want **refunded to you.** If Form 8888 is attached, check here . ▶☐ 73a

▶ b Routing number ▶ c Type: ☐ Checking ☐ Savings

▶ d Account number

74 Amount of line 72 you want **applied to your 2010 estimated tax** ▶ 74

Amount You Owe

75 **Amount you owe.** Subtract line 71 from line 60. For details on how to pay, see page 74 . ▶ 75

76 Estimated tax penalty (see page 74) . . . 76

Third Party Designee Do you want to allow another person to discuss this return with the IRS (see page 75)? ☐ **Yes.** Complete the following. ☐ **No**

Designee's name ▶ Phone no. ▶ Personal identification number (PIN) ▶

Sign Here
Joint return? See page 15. Keep a copy for your records.

Under penalties of perjury, I declare that I have examined this return and accompanying schedules and statements, and to the best of my knowledge and belief, they are true, correct, and complete. Declaration of preparer (other than taxpayer) is based on all information of which preparer has any knowledge.

Your signature | Date | Your occupation | Daytime phone number

Spouse's signature. If a joint return, **both** must sign. | Date | Spouse's occupation

Paid Preparer's Use Only

Preparer's signature ▶ | Date | Check if self-employed ☐ | Preparer's SSN or PTIN

Firm's name (or yours if self-employed), address, and ZIP code ▶ | EIN | Phone no.

Form **1040** (2009)

Fig 7-5 Sample Form 1040, page 2.

payments made for the tax year, and your W-2 wage withholding are reported here as well. Income tax liability is calculated based on these entries.

Property tax deduction

Home mortgage interest deduction

Other job expenses—enter job-related expenses as a W-2 wage employee

Total Schedule A itemized deductions—compare to standard deduction on Form 1040

SCHEDULE A (Form 1040) | **Itemized Deductions** | OMB No. 1545-0074 | **2009**

Department of the Treasury Internal Revenue Service (99) | ▶ Attach to Form 1040. ▶ See Instructions for Schedule A (Form 1040). | Attachment Sequence No. 07

Name(s) shown on Form 1040 | **Your social security number**

Section	Line	Description	Box	Total
Medical and Dental Expenses		**Caution.** Do not include expenses reimbursed or paid by others.		
	1	Medical and dental expenses (see page A-1)	1	
	2	Enter amount from Form 1040, line 38 [2]		
	3	Multiply line 2 by 7.5% (.075)	3	
	4	Subtract line 3 from line 1. If line 3 is more than line 1, enter -0-		4
Taxes You Paid (See page A-2.)	5	State and local **(check only one box):** a ☐ Income taxes, **or** b ☐ General sales taxes	5	
	6	Real estate taxes (see page A-5)	6	
	7	New motor vehicle taxes from line 11 of the worksheet on back. Skip this line if you checked box 5b	7	
	8	Other taxes. List type and amount ▶	8	
	9	Add lines 5 through 8		9
Interest You Paid (See page A-6.)	10	Home mortgage interest and points reported to you on Form 1098	10	
Note. Personal interest is not deductible.	11	Home mortgage interest not reported to you on Form 1098. If paid to the person from whom you bought the home, see page A-7 and show that person's name, identifying no., and address ▶	11	
	12	Points not reported to you on Form 1098. See page A-7 for special rules	12	
	13	Qualified mortgage insurance premiums (see page A-7)	13	
	14	Investment interest. Attach Form 4952 if required. (See page A-8.)	14	
	15	Add lines 10 through 14		15
Gifts to Charity If you made a gift and got a benefit for it, see page A-8.	16	Gifts by cash or check. If you made any gift of $250 or more, see page A-8	16	
	17	Other than by cash or check. If any gift of $250 or more, see page A-8. You **must** attach Form 8283 if over $500	17	
	18	Carryover from prior year	18	
	19	Add lines 16 through 18		19
Casualty and Theft Losses	20	Casualty or theft loss(es). Attach Form 4684. (See page A-10.)		20
Job Expenses and Certain Miscellaneous Deductions (See page A-10.)	21	Unreimbursed employee expenses—job travel, union dues, job education, etc. Attach Form 2106 or 2106-EZ if required. (See page A-10.) ▶	21	
	22	Tax preparation fees	22	
	23	Other expenses—investment, safe deposit box, etc. List type and amount ▶	23	
	24	Add lines 21 through 23	24	
	25	Enter amount from Form 1040, line 38 [25]		
	26	Multiply line 25 by 2% (.02)	26	
	27	Subtract line 26 from line 24. If line 26 is more than line 24, enter -0-		27
Other Miscellaneous Deductions	28	Other—from list on page A-11. List type and amount ▶		28
Total Itemized Deductions	29	Is Form 1040, line 38, over $166,800 (over $83,400 if married filing separately)? ☐ **No.** Your deduction is not limited. Add the amounts in the far right column for lines 4 through 28. Also, enter this amount on Form 1040, line 40a. ☐ **Yes.** Your deduction may be limited. See page A-11 for the amount to enter. ▶		29
	30	If you elect to itemize deductions even though they are less than your standard deduction, check here ▶ ☐		

For Paperwork Reduction Act Notice, see Form 1040 instructions. Cat. No. 17145C **Schedule A (Form 1040) 2009**

Fig 7-6 Sample Schedule A—Itemized Deductions.

Schedule A

Schedule A–Itemized Deductions (Fig 7-6) tabulates personal expense deductions such as medical expenses, state and local income taxes paid, real estate taxes paid, mortgage interest, and gifts to charity.

Form 1099-MISC

Income of $600 or more earned for services as an independent contractor dentist is reported to the IRS on Form 1099-MISC.

Income of $600 or more earned for services as an independent contractor dentist is reported to the IRS on Form 1099-MISC. Independent contractors pay quarterly estimated state and federal income tax, and they pay the entire amount of the Social Security and Medicare contribution (calculated on Schedule SE). Alternatively, independent contractor dentists may report their taxable income from those services on a Schedule C as a separate business entity. This Schedule C is then appended to their Form 1040.

Income Tax Bracket

income tax bracket
The tax rate expressed as a percentage on the last dollar of taxable income.

effective tax rate
Actual rate of taxes paid expressed as a percentage.

An income tax bracket is a way of visualizing the tax impact on your earned income. Dentists usually occupy the higher tax brackets. The highest federal tax bracket for 2009 was 35% (Box 7-4). Your stated income tax bracket is based on your last dollar earned; for example, earning $100,000 of taxable income in 2009 is referred to as being in the 28% tax bracket. Be aware, however, that you are only taxed a given rate on the amount of dollars that you have in that bracket. So, if you earned $8,360 in 2009, $8,350 would be taxed at 10%, and $10 would be taxed at 15%. The tax rate calculated based on your actual taxes paid is called the effective tax rate. Box 7-5 shows that the actual taxes paid on a $100,000 income would come to $21,720. This means that the effective tax rate is approximately 22% rather than 28%.

Tax Preparation

Checkbook software programs often can import data directly into tax preparation software. Individuals with uncomplicated tax returns sometimes elect to prepare their own tax returns using software programs rather than accountants or professional preparers. Tax preparation software takes the user through a sequence of steps, using an interview format and often incorporating icons and popup text boxes that explain tax issues in plain English. It groups relevant tax issues together and tax questions into a margin so you don't forget about them if or when you consult with an accountant or tax preparer.

Be ready to substantiate and defend each line item in your return because you may get audited. Retain all supporting documentation for 5 to 7 years.

Whichever way you choose to prepare your income tax return, be ready to substantiate and defend each line item because you can be–and

Box 7-4 Income tax brackets for a single taxpayer (2009)

Taxable income	Tax bracket
$0 to $8,350	10%
$8,350 to $33,950	15%
$33,950 to $82,250	25%
$82,250 to $171,550	28%
$171,550 to $372,950	33%
$372,950 and above	35%

Box 7-5 Calculation of actual taxes paid on a $100,000 taxable income

Taxable amount	Tax rate		Tax
$8,350 – $0 = $8,350	× 10%	=	$835
$33,950 – $8,350 = $25,600	× 15%	=	$3,840
$82,250 – $33,950 = $48,300	× 25%	=	$12,075
$100,000 – $82,250 = $17,750	× 28%	=	$4,970
	Tax due		$21,720

may get–audited. Retain and store all supporting invoices, receipts, checks, statements, and forms for approximately 5 to 7 years.

Some income tax documents to retain include:

- W-2s for wages earned
- Forms reporting interest and dividend income received from banks, financial institutions, etc
- Forms reporting interest and principal paid on loans such as student, mortgage, and car
- Bank statements
- Credit card statements
- Invoices: Supply, equipment, contractor
- Receipts for personal and business expense
- Log of business travel expenses

For more tips, go to the IRS website, which provides information to small businesses, the self-employed, and independent contractors. It is also prudent to seek professional advice from an attorney, accountant, or

tax preparer for information on business and tax structure, records systems, tax preparation, and reporting issues. But remember that, in the end, professionals may give advice and counsel, but you make the final decision and shoulder the consequences. You don't have to be an expert in taxes, but you should at least be literate.

Tax-Favored Savings Accounts

Every new dentist should open a tax-favored plan immediately after graduation. A small investment today can yield huge dividends over the years until retirement.

Every new dentist should open a tax-favored plan immediately after graduation. Delay short-term gratification from two martinis a month to invest in a plan. Time is an ally, and compound interest is magic. Thirty dollars–the cost of two martinis in Beverly Hills–invested at the beginning of a career grows tremendously in 25 years. Everyone is aware that income following graduation is notoriously unreliable, and the need to acquire life's necessities is high. Buy what you need, but try to put aside a few dollars every month in a rainy day fund. The tax-favored plan that invests pretax dollars to grow tax-free is a government gift. Following are some examples of tax-favored plans currently available.

Health Savings Account

An HSA is the best day-after-graduation plan. In 2009, an individual could contribute up to $3,000 tax-free annually to a single plan. It's a pretax deposit. There's also no tax taken when the money is withdrawn if that money is used to pay for a qualified health care expense. It's money that's tax-free when it goes into the account and tax-free when taken out of the account–absolute magic! You own and control the money in your HSA. As mentioned in chapter 5, an HSA must be paired with a high-deductible health plan, which in 2009 was medical insurance with a deductible of at least $1,050 for individuals and $2,100 for a family.

The HSA is designed to cover the gap between the first dollar expense and the deductible. Any money not used for a medical expense remains in the HSA to grow tax-free. For a young, healthy dentist, a high-deductible medical insurance makes sense because he or she is less likely to need ex-

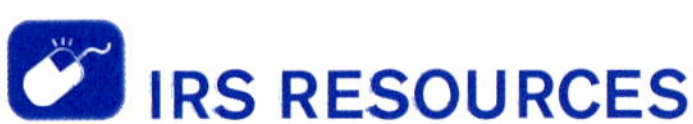

- www.irs.gov/businesses/small/index.html
- www.irs.gov/businesses/small/article/0,,id=115041,00.html
- www.irs.gov/businesses/small/article/0,,id=179115,00.html

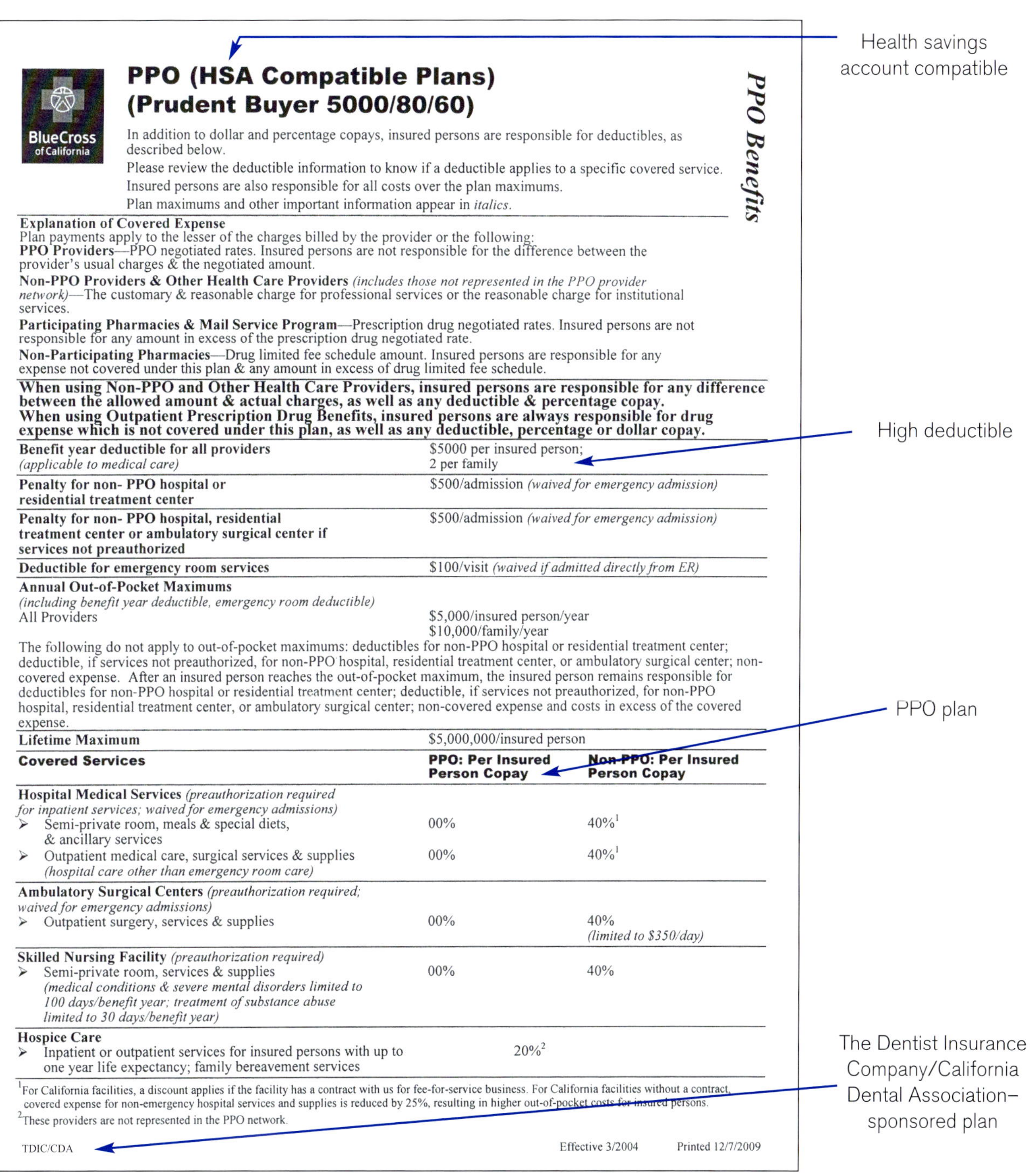

BlueCross of California

PPO (HSA Compatible Plans) (Prudent Buyer 5000/80/60)

PPO Benefits

In addition to dollar and percentage copays, insured persons are responsible for deductibles, as described below.

Please review the deductible information to know if a deductible applies to a specific covered service.

Insured persons are also responsible for all costs over the plan maximums.

Plan maximums and other important information appear in *italics*.

Explanation of Covered Expense

Plan payments apply to the lesser of the charges billed by the provider or the following:

PPO Providers—PPO negotiated rates. Insured persons are not responsible for the difference between the provider's usual charges & the negotiated amount.

Non-PPO Providers & Other Health Care Providers *(includes those not represented in the PPO provider network)*—The customary & reasonable charge for professional services or the reasonable charge for institutional services.

Participating Pharmacies & Mail Service Program—Prescription drug negotiated rates. Insured persons are not responsible for any amount in excess of the prescription drug negotiated rate.

Non-Participating Pharmacies—Drug limited fee schedule amount. Insured persons are responsible for any expense not covered under this plan & any amount in excess of drug limited fee schedule.

When using Non-PPO and Other Health Care Providers, insured persons are responsible for any difference between the allowed amount & actual charges, as well as any deductible & percentage copay. When using Outpatient Prescription Drug Benefits, insured persons are always responsible for drug expense which is not covered under this plan, as well as any deductible, percentage or dollar copay.

Benefit year deductible for all providers *(applicable to medical care)*	$5000 per insured person; 2 per family
Penalty for non- PPO hospital or residential treatment center	$500/admission *(waived for emergency admission)*
Penalty for non- PPO hospital, residential treatment center or ambulatory surgical center if services not preauthorized	$500/admission *(waived for emergency admission)*
Deductible for emergency room services	$100/visit *(waived if admitted directly from ER)*
Annual Out-of-Pocket Maximums *(including benefit year deductible, emergency room deductible)* All Providers	$5,000/insured person/year $10,000/family/year

The following do not apply to out-of-pocket maximums: deductibles for non-PPO hospital or residential treatment center; deductible, if services not preauthorized, for non-PPO hospital, residential treatment center, or ambulatory surgical center; non-covered expense. After an insured person reaches the out-of-pocket maximum, the insured person remains responsible for deductibles for non-PPO hospital or residential treatment center; deductible, if services not preauthorized, for non-PPO hospital, residential treatment center, or ambulatory surgical center; non-covered expense and costs in excess of the covered expense.

Lifetime Maximum	$5,000,000/insured person

Covered Services	**PPO: Per Insured Person Copay**	**Non-PPO: Per Insured Person Copay**
Hospital Medical Services *(preauthorization required for inpatient services; waived for emergency admissions)*		
➢ Semi-private room, meals & special diets, & ancillary services	00%	40%[1]
➢ Outpatient medical care, surgical services & supplies *(hospital care other than emergency room care)*	00%	40%[1]
Ambulatory Surgical Centers *(preauthorization required; waived for emergency admissions)*		
➢ Outpatient surgery, services & supplies	00%	40% *(limited to $350/day)*
Skilled Nursing Facility *(preauthorization required)*		
➢ Semi-private room, services & supplies *(medical conditions & severe mental disorders limited to 100 days/benefit year; treatment of substance abuse limited to 30 days/benefit year)*	00%	40%
Hospice Care		
➢ Inpatient or outpatient services for insured persons with up to one year life expectancy; family bereavement services	20%[2]	

[1]For California facilities, a discount applies if the facility has a contract with us for fee-for-service business. For California facilities without a contract, covered expense for non-emergency hospital services and supplies is reduced by 25%, resulting in higher out-of-pocket costs for insured persons.

[2]These providers are not represented in the PPO network.

TDIC/CDA Effective 3/2004 Printed 12/7/2009

Fig 7-7 Sample high-deductible health plan.

pensive medical care, and the medical insurance premium is low. State dental associations offer high-deductible medical insurance plans and work with various HSA vendors (Fig 7-7).

Box 7-6 HSA and traditional IRA tax shield effect

	HSA only	HSA and IRA
Gross income	$125,000	$125,000
Standard deduction (single)	$5,700	$5,700
One exemption	$3,650	$3,650
Taxable income	$115,650	$115,650
Income tax (28% tax bracket)	$26,102	$26,102
HSA contribution	$3,000	$3,000
Traditional IRA	0	$5,000
Adjusted taxable income	$112,650	$107,650
Income tax (28% tax bracket)	$25,262	$23,862
Income tax savings	**$840**	**$2,240**

Traditional Individual Retirement Account (IRA)

traditional IRA
Personal retirement plan for which contributions, gains, interest, and dividends are tax-free until they are withdrawn. In addition, early withdrawal (ie, before you reach age 59 ½ years) results in a penalty fee.

The traditional IRA is a personal retirement plan. Contributions are invested tax-free (ie, you can deduct this amount on Form 1040). However, the deductibility of the traditional IRA contribution is subject to limitations based on your adjusted gross income for the year and whether you or your spouse is covered by an employer's retirement plan. Financial institutions offer a variety of IRA plans. Invested funds, gains, interest, and dividends accumulate tax-free until they are withdrawn, at which point they are then taxed. Early withdrawal (ie, before you reach age 59 ½ years) will result in a penalty fee. In 2009, contributions up to $5,000 could be made annually.

Box 7-6 shows that you can contribute $3,000 to an HSA and pay $840 less in federal income tax. This is the same as putting away only $2,160 to have a full $3,000 in your HSA. The full $3,000 HSA contribution is tax-free and can be withdrawn at any time–also tax-free–to pay for any qualified health care expense such as prescription eyeglasses. If you also contribute $5,000 to a traditional IRA, you will pay a total of $2,240 less in federal income tax. In other words, you can put aside $5,760 ($15.78 a day, about the cost of one martini in Beverly Hills) and Uncle Sam kicks in another $2,240 so that you have a total of $8,000 to put away.

Roth IRA

A Roth IRA is a personal retirement plan, and, for income tax–reporting purposes, it is the exact opposite of a traditional IRA. Roth contributions are made with after-tax dollars, which means that you pay the income tax on the money before you make the Roth IRA contribution. However, the funds, gains, interest, and dividends accumulate tax-free, and upon withdrawal the money is distributed tax-free, although penalties may apply for early withdrawal (ie, before you reach age 59 ½ years). To be eligible for the plan, for a single person adjusted gross income must be less than $120,000 with the phaseout starting at $105,000 and for a married couple adjusted gross income must be less than $176,000 with the phaseout starting at $166,000. This stipulation is not usually an issue for a recent graduate. In 2009 contributions were capped at $5,000 annually.

Roth IRA
Personal retirement plan for which contributions are made with after-tax dollars, but gains, interest, and dividends accumulate tax-free, and upon withdrawal the money is distributed tax-free, although penalties may apply for early withdrawal (ie, before you reach age 59 ½ years).

Simplified Employee Pension IRA

A simplified employee pension IRA (SEP-IRA) is an employer's retirement plan established by sole proprietors. It is used instead of a Keogh retirement plan because it has few tax filing requirements. In 2009, its annual contribution was capped at 20% of your net adjusted gross income or $49,000. Contributions are flexible and the amount can vary each year. SEP-IRA rules require that qualified employees be included, with an employer funding 100% of the employee's SEP-IRA contribution, up to 25% of the employee's earned income. The plan cannot be discriminatory in favor of the highly compensated, and contributions should be made for each employee. In 2009, an eligible employee had to be at least 21 years old with 3 years of service in the past 5 years, having earned at least $550 from the employer in the past year.

simplified employee pension IRA (SEP-IRA)
An employer's retirement plan established by sole proprietors. Employers must fund 100% of qualified employees' SEP-IRA contributions up to 25% of the employee's earned income.

Savings Incentive Match Plan for Employees IRA

A savings incentive match plan for employees IRA (SIMPLE-IRA) is an employer's retirement plan. Under a SIMPLE-IRA plan, employees and employers may make contributions to a traditional IRA set up for qualified employees and a sole proprietor. Employers can match an employee's contribution dollar-for-dollar, up to 3% of each employee's salary or elect a nonmatching contribution of 2% of each employee's salary compensation. The SIMPLE-IRA is suited as a startup retirement savings

savings incentive match plan for employees IRA (SIMPLE-IRA)
An employer's retirement plan in which employees and employers make contributions to a traditional IRA set up for qualified employees and a sole proprietor. Employers can match an employee's contribution dollar-for-dollar, up to 3% of each employee's salary, or elect a nonmatching contribution of 2% of each employee's salary compensation.

plan for a sole proprietor who wishes to offer a small retirement plan to employees.

Underfunding a Retirement Plan

Some business retirement plans such as an SEP require an employer to fund an eligible employee's retirement plan. Funding only the employer's retirement plan and not an eligible employee's plan can result in the disallowance of the entire plan and payment of back taxes, as well as interest and penalties. In a long-standing retirement plan the dollar amount of sanctions can be potentially staggering.

A Word on Words

Following are some important but often confused terms. Most of them have already been covered elsewhere in this chapter or in another chapter in the book, but the concepts are important enough to bear repeating here.

- *Revenue versus Income: Revenue* is the money that's received directly from a patient or insurance company, whereas *income* is money that remains after expenses are paid.
- *Production versus Collection: Production* counts the dollar when it is earned, eg, when a procedure is completed. *Collection* counts the dollar when it is deposited in your bank account. Think of production as accrual accounting and collection as cash accounting.
- *Accounts receivable: Accounts receivable* is the arithmetic difference between production and collection. It sits on the books until collected. It is a paper entry only–it can't buy a cup of coffee. *Accounts receivable turnover* measures the speed in which payment is received and money is deposited into your bank account. *Aging accounts receivable* measures how long payment has been outstanding.
- *Average versus Margin: Average* and *margin* are two distinct ways of looking at finances. We report in averages, but we live on the margin. We might average $30,000 in revenue per month, $20,000 in expense per month, and $10,000 in income every month. However, in any given month, the rent might be due on the 1st, salaries paid on the 1st and 15th, and laboratory expense paid on the 20th. In that same month, insurance checks might arrive on a Friday and patient payments around

the 30th. So, on the margin, considerably more income is earned on the last day than the first day. A similar situation occurs when yearly averages are applied to weekly or monthly revenue and expenses. What this means to a growing practice is that you must plan for extreme cash flow fluctuations in a specific period, whether it be a week, month, or quarter.

- *Market share versus Profitability: Market share* does not equal *profitability.* A large patient base and high revenue do not necessarily equate to higher income. Fees may not be commensurate with overhead. The marginal revenue from an additional patient might not equal or exceed the marginal cost to render the treatment.
- *Depreciate versus Expense:* To *depreciate* a tangible asset like dental equipment is to write down the value over a period of years. To *expense* dental equipment is to immediately write down the entire value in the same year it is purchased, which is the fastest depreciation method available. Both are important tax shield strategies and noncash bookkeeping entries. Expensing reduces tax liability for that year to shield other income, but then the tax shield is not available in subsequent years even though loan payments continue. Finding the proper balance between depreciation, expensing, income, and loan payments is desirable but elusive.
- *Discount versus Compound: Discount* is to calculating the present value as *compound* is to calculating the future value. Both use the same modified formula but calculate values moving in opposite directions in time. The rate of discount (or compounding if going forward) is the expected rate of return from investments with similar risk and financial leverage (ie, loan interest versus return). There is no standard discount rate for any given investment, which means that determining a discount rate for any investment is more of a financial art than an economic science.

References

1. Practice start-up loans from Bank of America. Bank of America website. http://www.bankofamerica.com/small_business/practicesolutions/index.cfm?template=new_practice_startups. Accessed 29 December 2009.
2. What is an SBA loan: Excel National Bank. Excel National Bank website. http://www.bankexcel.com/home/lending/sba/what. Accessed 29 December 2009.
3. Dental practice acquisition and start up financing–Financing programs–Dentists–Matsco. Matsco website. http://www.matsco.com/dentists/practice-financing-programs/practice-start-up-financing.htm. Accessed 29 December 2009.

4. Conkey C. How to boost your credit score: Increasingly, employers, others check your ranking; do you really need that store card? Wall Street Journal. November 19, 2005. http://online.wsj.com/article/SB113236756411202164.html. Accessed 29 December 2009.
5. Pilon M. Time to step up for credit score: A higher number is needed for some loans; how to improve your chances. The Wall Street Journal. January 2, 2009.

Complying with Dental Practice Regulations

Michael Okuji, DDS, MPH, MBA

This chapter brings together dental practice registration, regulations, and compliance issues into a single source, but it's not meant to be exhaustive. Rather, it provides guidance on the first steps toward managing a private practice. Regulations are designed and enacted to benefit and protect the public, employees, and patients. Regulatory compliance is overseen and enforced by federal, state, and local agencies. Disregard, misapplication, or noncompliance may result in penalties and remediation. In past generations, the safety of the patient and employee was left to the discretion and judgment of the dentist. Nevermore.

Disregard, misapplication, or noncompliance to regulations may result in penalties and remediation.

The dentist as business owner, employer, taxpayer, facility manager, and health care professional is challenged to appropriately apply myriad rules that can be common sense or arcane. The onus to understand, apply, and enforce the pertinent regulation rests squarely on the sole proprietor.

This chapter is divided into sections on: personal registration, employer reporting, and dental office regulatory compliance. For the purpose of illustration, some specific examples are given for the state of California and the city and county of San Francisco. It is the reader's responsibility to research individual state and local regulations.

The chapter is by no means a complete compilation of every regulation that you need to comply with, nor is it completely current–regulations can change daily. Instead, it's meant to introduce you to the environment in which you will practice and equip you with the basic knowledge you need to move toward your first day of private practice. You will need to refer to official sources of published regulations, detailed compliance manuals, and, if needed, professional assistance in each category.

Personal Registration

Licensure

Obtaining a dental license is the first order of business for the new graduate.

Dental licensure is regulated by every US state. Obtaining a dental license is the first order of business for the new graduate. Licensure can be by examination, residency, or credential. Graduation from dental school makes you eligible to sit for the appropriate examination and then apply for a state dental license. Many states offer licensure after successfully completing an approved 1-year Advanced Education in General Dentistry (AEGD) program or the general practice residency (GPR) program without taking a licensing examination. Remember that licensure by credentials doesn't apply to first-time applicants (see chapter 1).

An application form, fingerprinting, and fees may apply. In addition, an examination that covers the state's specific dental practice act and dental ethics may be required. Since licensure isn't uniform among states, you should contact the state where you plan to practice for details.

The Dental Board of California accepts scores from the California or the Western Regional Examining Board (WREB) examination for licensure. For first-time applicants, California issues a license upon completion of a 12-month GPR or AEGD residency. All new licensees have to pass the California law and ethics examination, complete an application, submit to fingerprinting, and pay fees. The dental license is issued on a biennial basis (ie, once every 2 years).

Fictitious Name Permit

The Dental Board of California issues a fictitious name permit, which is required to practice under an assumed name (eg, Pacific Ocean Dental). This permit is distinct and separate from any requirement that a city government may impose. Note that a fictitious name permit is not required if you practice under your name, eg, Michael Okuji, DDS, or Dr Michael Okuji, General Dentistry.

Other Special Permits

The Dental Board of California issues permits for performing specific treatments, including conscious sedation, oral conscious sedation, oral conscious sedation on minors, oral and maxillofacial surgery, general anesthesia, and elective facial cosmetic surgery.

Drug License

In order to prescribe controlled drugs, you must apply for a federal Drug Enforcement Administration (DEA) registration number, which can be done online. Fill out a new applicant Form 224 for practitioners. You must have a tax identification number or social security number (SSN), state controlled substance registration, and state dental license information, as well as a credit card to pay the fee.

The DEA number is issued on a biennial basis. It is required to prescribe Schedule II drugs (eg, oxycodone); Schedule III drugs (eg, hydrocodone); and Schedule IV drugs (eg, diazepam). The DEA registration number is imprinted on state-approved, tamper-resistant prescription forms along with the state dental license number. Pharmacies require a DEA registration number and state dental license number to prescribe drugs by telephone.

Prescription Pad

California dentists order tamper-resistant forms from security prescription printer companies that are preapproved by the California Board of Pharmacy and the Department of Justice. The California Attorney General's Office publishes a directory listing of these companies, which is updated when a new security prescription printer company is approved. A California state license number and a copy of the DEA registration are required to place the order.

Radiation Safety Certificate

In California, a dentist or employee must pass a dental board–approved radiation safety course prior to exposing any radiographs, and the Committee on Dental Auxiliaries is notified of each person's successful completion of the required course to record compliance. Auxiliaries certified

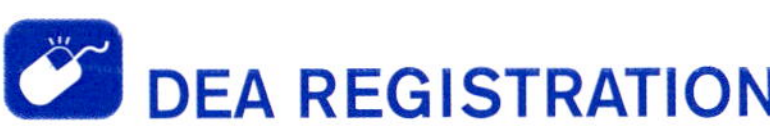

- www.deadiversion.usdoj.gov/drugreg/reg_apps/onlineforms_new.htm

in radiation safety may operate dental radiographic equipment under the general supervision of a dentist.

National Provider Identifier Number

national provider identifiers (NPIs) Unique identification numbers that are used when submitting dental claims; also called *dental insurance provider numbers.*

The National Plan and Provider Enumeration System (NPPES) assigns national provider identifiers (NPIs), which are unique identification numbers that are used when submitting claims. They are also called *dental insurance provider numbers.* You can apply for an NPI online.

Dental reimbursement plans require the NPI on claim forms, and dental plans and electronic claims clearinghouses use the NPI for administrative and financial transactions specified by the Health Insurance Portability and Accountability Act (HIPAA), including electronic claims and digital radiographs.

Employer Reporting

Employer Identification Number

employer identification number (EIN) Identifies employers to the Social Security Administration (SSA) and the Internal Revenue Service (IRS) and tracks federal income tax withholding and SSA documents; also called the *federal tax identification.*

As an employer, you must obtain a federal employer identification number (EIN), also called the *federal tax identification,* which will identify you to the Social Security Administration (SSA) and the Internal Revenue Service (IRS). It is distinctly different from your SSN and NPI. The EIN tracks federal income tax withholding and SSA documents (eg, Federal Insurance Contributions Act [FICA] and Medicare), and it's required for every business that has employees. You can obtain an EIN by filing Form SS-4 or by registering online, which is a free service and results in the immediate issuance of an EIN. The EIN webpage also has links for specific states, which you can use to obtain a state employer number. California requires employers to have a state employer number.

NPI APPLICATION/EIN APPLICATION

- https://nppes.cms.hhs.gov/NPPES
- www.irs.gov/businesses/small/article/0,,id=98350,00.html

Table 8-1 2009 federal tax withholdings*

Withholding	Employer amount (% of wages)	Employee amount (% of wages)
Income tax	0.00	Variable*
FICA	6.20	6.20
Medicare	1.45	1.45
Unemployment tax	0.08†	0.00

*See Publication 15, Circular E.
†On the first $7,000 for each employee.

Table 8-2 2009 California state tax withholdings

Withholding	Payee	Amount (% of wages)
State income tax	Employee	Variable*
State disability insurance	Employee	1.1
Unemployment insurance	Employer	1.5†
Employment training tax	Employer	0.1†

*Calculated using tax table.
†On the first $7,000 for each employee.

Withholdings

An employer must withhold federal and state taxes from employee wages. Federal withholdings include the federal income tax and FICA withholding, which funds Social Security and Medicare (Table 8-1). An employer matches employee FICA and Medicare contributions dollar for dollar.

An employer withholds state income tax and state disability insurance from employee wages and, in California, pays unemployment insurance and employment training tax on behalf of its employees (Table 8-2).

Employee withholding is regularly reported and paid using several different federal and state forms (see following sections on wage forms), which can be time consuming. Reports and payments can be due monthly, quarterly, or annually. A dentist with only a few employees usually documents, files, and makes the payments, whereas a dentist with a large staff may designate a bookkeeper or outsource the process to a payroll company.

Reporting and paying employee withholdings is a time-consuming process; dentists with more than just a few employees often opt to delegate the job to a bookkeeper or outsource the process to a payroll company.

Federal Employer Wage Forms

Federal employment eligibility verification (Form I-9)

Every new employee fills out a federal employment eligibility verification (Form I-9), documenting that he or she (whether a citizen or noncitizen) is authorized to work in the United States. The form is kept in the office and not filed with the US Citizenship and Immigrations Service or any government agency. There is no fee for the form.

Employee's withholding allowance certificate (Form W-4)

Each employee fills out an employee's withholding allowance certificate (W-4) when he or she first starts work, declaring marital status and the number of eligible allowances for federal tax withholding purposes. A new W-4 is filled out each time an existing employee changes his or her number of allowances and/or marital status, and the form is kept in the office.

Wage and tax statement (Form W-2)

The wage and tax statement (W-2) is issued annually for each employee who was paid a wage for the tax year. A copy is filed with the SSA by March 2nd (March 31st for employers who file electronically) in the year following the wage reporting. If you don't file electronically, paper forms must be machine-readable (not downloadable). Total wages reported to the SSA on Form W-2 must equal the wage reported to the IRS on Schedule C of the Form 1040 personal tax return.

There are several copies of the Form W-2, and each is designated for a specific party:

- Copy A is filed with the SSA.
- Copy B is for the employee's federal tax form.
- Copy C is for the employee's records.
- Copy D is for the employer.

FEDERAL EMPLOYER WAGE FORMS

- I-9: www.uscis.gov/files/form/I-9.pdf
- W-4: www.irs.gov/pub/irs-pdf/fw4.pdf
- W-2: www.irs.gov/pub/irs-pdf/fw2.pdf
- W-3: www.irs.gov/pub/irs-pdf/fw3.pdf
- Publication 15, Circular E: www.irs.gov/pub/irs-pdf/p15.pdf
- Form 1099-MISC: www.irs.gov/pub/irs-pdf/f1099msc.pdf

- Copy 1 is for employer's state tax department.
- Copy 2 is for employees' state income tax return.

Federal employer's transmittal of wage and tax statement (Form W-3)

The federal employer's transmittal of wage and tax statement (Form W-3) is filed annually with the SSA. Copy A of each of the employer's W-2s is attached; the form is never filed alone. The form can be submitted electronically or in paper form, but paper forms must be machine-readable (not downloadable). As with Form W-2, total wages reported to the SSA on Form W-3 must equal the wage reported to the IRS on Schedule C of the Form 1040 personal tax return.

Federal employer's tax guide (Publication 15, Circular E)

The federal employer's tax guide (Publication 15, Circular E) calculates, in tabular form, how much federal income tax to withhold from an employee's wages. This is accomplished by first selecting a page by marital status (single or married) and pay period (daily, weekly, biweekly, or semimonthly), then scanning across the top of the page for the number of allowances declared on the W-4, and finally scrolling down the side of the page to the gross wages paid in the period. The number at the intersection of the appropriate column and row is the amount of federal income tax that should be withheld from gross wages and paid to the SSA every month on Form 8190.

Federal tax deposit coupons (Form 8109-B)

The federal tax deposit coupons (Form 8109-B) are used to report the federal income tax, FICA, and Medicare that is withheld from employee wages plus the employer's contribution to FICA and Medicare on behalf of the employee. The Form 8109-B coupon and payment should be deposited at your bank each month.

Employer's quarterly federal tax return (Form 941)

The employer's quarterly federal tax return (Form 941) summarizes and reconciles employee total wages, employee deductions, and the employer contribution that was paid during the quarter through Form 8109-B. Over- or underpayment can be reconciled here.

Employer's annual federal unemployment tax return (Form 940)

The employer's annual federal unemployment tax return (FUTA; Form 940) reports your yearly federal unemployment contribution, which applies to the first $7,000 paid to each employee during a calendar year. Both FUTA and the state unemployment tax provide funds to pay unemployment compensation to workers who have lost their job. Only employers pay this tax.

Form 1099-MISC

Form 1099-MISC is issued to independent contractors to report earnings of more than $600 to the IRS. Independent contractors pay the income tax and the full FICA contribution; there is no employer contribution.

State Employer Wage Forms (California)

Withholding and reporting documentation varies from state to state, so be sure to research what is required in your state.

In addition to the federal requirements, state withholding and reporting documentation must be processed. Every state is slightly different; California is used here as an example.

In California, the Employment Development Department (EDD) tabulates and collects employee wage deductions and monitors employment practices.

State employer account number

The state employer account number is separate and distinct from the federal EIN. In California, it can be obtained online, through the mail, or by phone.

Payroll tax deposit coupon (Form DE-88)

The payroll tax deposit coupon (Form DE-88) summarizes and reconciles employee state income tax and state disability insurance withholding from employee wages and the employer contribution for unemployment insurance and the employment training tax. Those payments are submitted directly to EDD with a completed Form DE-88. In most cases, these payments are made quarterly. A 10% penalty plus interest is assessed on late payments.

Quarterly wage and withholding report (Form DE-6)

The quarterly wage and withholding report (Form DE-6) is the quarterly wage report to the state that declares all employee wage and withholding. No money is sent with this form; payment is made using Form DE-88.

Annual reconciliation statement (Form DE-7)

The annual reconciliation statement (Form DE-7) reconciles wages paid and withholdings for the calendar year, and it's due by January 31st for the previous calendar year. No money should be sent with this report.

Report of new employee(s) (Form DE-34)

The report of new employee(s) (DE-34) is a quarterly report sent to the state that lists all the new employees you've hired.

Report of independent contractors (Form 542)

The report of independent contractors (Form 542), which is sent to the state, lists the income paid to an independent contractor (ie, where no taxes are withheld).

Workers' Compensation Insurance

Workers' compensation insurance, as discussed in chapter 5, is state-mandated insurance that covers employees for any on-the-job injury or illness, no matter who is at fault. In return, the employee is prevented from suing the employer over the injuries. California employers are required by law to have workers' compensation insurance, even if they have only one employee. Employers pay for workers' compensation insurance on behalf of their workers. If a disagreement arises over issues such as whether the injury was sustained on the job, it is resolved through the Division of Workers' Compensation or before a judge at a local office.

Some state dental associations, including the California Dental Association, offer a number of workers' compensation insurance products to its members.

Disability Insurance

As described in chapter 5, state disability insurance is an employee program that provides partial wage replacement to workers who are unable to work because of pregnancy or a non–job-related injury or illness. State disability insurance is separate and distinct from any private disability policy.

A pregnant employee is eligible for state disability insurance benefits for up to 4 weeks before her expected delivery date and up to 6 weeks after the delivery in a normal pregnancy, but a physician may certify a longer period if the delivery is by cesarean section.

Paid family leave

Paid family leave is a program provided by California that provides up to 6 weeks of benefits for individuals who must take time off to care for a seriously ill child, spouse, parent, or registered domestic partner or to bond with a newborn baby, adopted child, or foster child. Workers who participate in the California state disability program are entitled to paid family leave.

Unemployment Insurance

unemployment insurance
Nationwide program created to provide partial wage replacement to unemployed workers while they conduct an active search for new work.

Unemployment insurance is a nationwide program created to provide partial wage replacement to unemployed workers while they conduct an active search for new work. It is based on federal law and executed through state law. Employers finance the program through FUTA and state contributions.

Minimum Wage

Minimum wage is determined by each state. The California minimum wage law covers nearly all employees in California. However, there is an exception in which workers can be paid no less than 85% of the minimum wage during their first 160 hours of employment in an occupation in which they have no previous similar or related experience.

Overtime

Overtime pay is calculated at one and one-half times the regular rate of pay for hours in excess of 8 hours, up to 12 hours in any workday, and for the first 8 hours worked on the 7th consecutive day. It is calculated per day, not on a 40-hour workweek, which means that it can impact the wage base for those who work 10-hour days for 4 consecutive days.

Double time is paid for hours in excess of 12 hours in any workday and for all hours in excess of 8 hours on the 7th consecutive day.

Dental Office Regulatory Compliance

Dental office regulations are designed to protect the health and safety of employees and patients. You should prepare for dental office regulatory compliance before you open your doors. Regulatory compliance requires continuous, regular, and meticulous maintenance of records, and continual employee training is mandatory. Each mandate comes with a protocol for implementation, inspection, enforcement, and penalties for noncompliance. Although a dentist needs to know the regulatory requirements and implement the protocols, the end managerial goal is to skillfully delegate this enormous responsibility to a key office staff member or to outsource its management.

Although a dentist needs to know the regulatory requirements and implement the protocols, the end managerial goal is to skillfully delegate this enormous responsibility to a key office staff member or to outsource its management.

Regulatory mandates come from federal, state, and local agencies, and, individually, they are manageable; however, in aggregate, they are burdensome and baffling. Disgruntled employees are a major source of inspection requests. Employees usually know every rule and regulation and what agency is responsible to enforce each, so there are no secrets and no hidden corners in the dental office. Therefore, you should be conversant–if not expert–in the regulations that affect your office and practice, including those issues that are idiosyncratic to your location. California and San Francisco will be used as examples for regulatory compliance at the state and local levels, respectively.

You should be conversant—if not expert—in the regulations that affect your office and practice, including those issues that are idiosyncratic to your location.

Federal Regulatory Compliance

Regulations and regulatory agencies are designed to protect the patient, employee, and the public at large. HIPAA is a federal agency designated to protect the privacy of patients, and the Occupational Safety and Health Administration (OSHA) is a federal agency designated to protect the health and safety of employees.

Health Insurance Portability and Accountability Act (HIPAA)

HIPAA was enacted to protect the privacy of patient health information. It applies to dentists who conduct transactions in electronic form such as electronic claims submission, dispersal of digital radiographs, and Internet benefit eligibility inquiries. If you transmit claims electronically, HIPAA requires that you obtain an NPI number, and some dental plans require a NPI number on paper claims as well.

HIPAA was enacted to protect the privacy of patient health information.

In addition, HIPAA requires that your patients have a right to:

- See and get a copy of their health record within 30 days
- Have corrections made to their health information
- Receive notice on their first visit that tells them how their health information is being used and shared
- Decide whether to give their permission, in writing, before their information can be used or shared for certain purposes
- Receive a report on when and why their health information is shared
- Ask to be contacted somewhere other than their home
- Ask that their information not be shared
- File a complaint if they believe their information was used or shared in a way not allowed under the privacy law
- File a complaint if they were not informed of their right to file a complaint at all

The privacy notice they receive from you will provide them with information about who to talk to in your office and how to file a complaint. They can also file a complaint with the federal government.

Dentists must be compliant with HIPAA to ensure patient privacy and security. In accordance with privacy rules, a dentist must:

- Provide a privacy notice to each patient.
- Adopt and implement privacy procedures.
- Train employees so they understand the privacy procedures.
- Secure patient records (see below).
- Designate an individual to enforce the privacy procedures.

Security rules the dentist must follow include:

- Patient records that are created and stored on computers must remain confidential.
- Administrative policies must be instituted to safeguard electronic records.
- All office personnel should be trained in these security measures.

You and your staff will need to know how HIPAA privacy and security mandates apply to your practice and exactly how to implement the measures.

You and your staff will need to know how all these issues apply to your practice and exactly how to implement the measures. The first and best resource for integrating HIPAA privacy and security mandates in your office is the *HIPAA Privacy Kit* manual and CD-ROM available from the

Box 8-1 Examples of issues requiring written plans and record keeping under OSHA

Written plans:
- Disease transmission
- Blood-borne pathogens rule
- Exposure control plan
- Postexposure management
- Hazardous waste management
- Hazard communication
- Ergonomics
- Fire and emergency

Record keeping:
- Schedule and method implementation
- Employee medical record form (hepatitis B)
- Informed refusal for hepatitis B vaccination
- Identification, evaluation, and selection of engineering and work practice controls
- Housekeeping schedule
- Sharps injury log
- Individual training documentation
- Employee accident/bodily fluid exposure and follow-up
- Confirmation of source patient's denial for testing
- Employee-informed refusal of postexposure medical evaluation
- Checklist for exposure follow-up requirements
- Written opinion of a health care evaluator

American Dental Association (ADA). Or you can turn to a consultant; the intricacy of HIPAA compliance has led to the development of numerous consultant businesses that can set up and maintain a system of compliance for you.

Occupational Safety and Health Administration (OSHA)

OSHA is a federal worker's safety agency that mandates a safe and healthy workplace for employees by setting and enforcing standards. A valuable resource for OSHA compliance is the ADA's workbook and DVD set *OSHA Training for Dental Professionals.*

OSHA is a federal worker's safety agency that mandates a safe and healthy workplace for employees by setting and enforcing standards.

In California, the state OSHA enforcement agency is called Cal/OSHA. Many California mandates are more stringent than the federal mandates.

OSHA addresses many issues in the dental office, including mundane yet important concerns like proper exit signs and fire extinguishers. OSHA compliance requires that you have both written plans and record keeping in place for specified issues. Complete descriptions and implementation procedures for each of the written plan and record keeping requirements are beyond the scope of this book; however, some examples are given in Box 8-1.

State Regulatory Compliance (California)

Radiation machine registration

California requires that each x-ray tube be registered, and the x-ray machine must be registered within 30 days of its acquisition. This is the dentist's responsibility; the dental equipment supplier cannot register x-ray machines.

Air compressor permit

Nearly all air compressors require a permit, so be sure to check with your dental equipment supplier when you purchase and install a new air compressor.

Hazardous waste identification number

A federal EPA ID number is required to dispose of hazardous waste, which includes amalgam, traps and filters that contain amalgam, fixer, developer, lead film foil, and chemical sterilizer fluid.

A federal Environmental Protection Agency identification (EPA ID) number is required to dispose of hazardous waste, which includes amalgam, traps and filters that contain amalgam, fixer, developer, lead film foil, and chemical sterilizer fluid. You're also required to have an EPA ID number if your practice generates more than 1 kg per month of Resource Conservation and Recovery Act (RCRA) acutely hazardous waste or more than 100 kg per month of other RCRA waste. There is an exemption if less waste is generated and other requirements are met. Exempt offices are called *conditionally exempt small quantity generators.* Because California doesn't have an equivalent exemption, nearly all offices in the state that generate hazardous waste and don't have a federal EPA ID must have a California EPA ID.

Medical waste registration

Dentists who generate medical waste, such as needles and other sharps and biohazard materials, must register with their local or state enforcement agency. To protect the public and the environment from infectious exposure to disease-causing agents, the California Medical Waste Management Program in the Environmental Management Branch regulates the generation, handling, storage, treatment, and disposal of medical waste.

Dental materials fact sheet

The Dental Board of California develops, distributes, and administers a user-friendly dental materials fact sheet (DMFS) that should be given to patients before any restorative work is begun. It applies to all offices, even those that do not use silver amalgam, and to all types of restorations, including crowns, bridges, inlays, and veneers of any composition. A den-

Box 8-2 Known carcinogens and/or reproductive toxicants*

- Mercury (silver amalgam)
- Beryllium
- Ceramic fibers
- Chloroform
- Chromium
- Crystalline silica
- Formaldehyde
- Methylene chloride
- Nickel (associated with nonamalgam fillings)
- Toluene (root canal materials, impression materials, sealants)

*As determined by the government of California.

tist is required to obtain a signed acknowledgement that the patient received the DMFS, and a copy of the acknowledgement must be placed in the patient's record. The form can be obtained from the Dental Board of California's website to copy and distribute as needed.

Following is a sample DMFS acknowledgement:

I, (patient's name), acknowledge I have received from (dentist's name) a copy of the dental materials fact sheet dated (month) (day), (year), as required by law.

(patient's signature) (date).

Proposition 65

California's Proposition 65 requires the governor to publish a list of chemicals that have been determined by the government of California to be known carcinogens and/or reproductive toxicants (Box 8-2).

Dental offices with nine or more employees are required to prominently post a Proposition 65 sign, and offices with fewer than nine employees are encouraged to post the sign. To comply, the language on the sign must strictly adhere to the wording developed by the California Dental Association (Fig 8-1), and the sign must be prominently placed in a location that gives patients the opportunity to receive a clear and reason able warning prior to any exposure. A single sign prominently displayed in the waiting room is deemed to be in compliance.

NOTICE TO PATIENTS
PROPOSITION 65 WARNING

- Dental amalgam, used in many fillings, causes exposure to mercury, a chemical known to the State of California to cause birth defects or other reproductive harm.
- Root canal treatments and restorations, including fillings, crowns, and bridges, use chemicals known to the State of California to cause cancer.
- The US Food and Drug Administration has studied the situation and approved for use all dental restorative materials.
- Consult with your dentist to determine which materials are appropriate for your treatment.

Fig 8-1 A Proposition 65 sign, which must be prominently displayed by all dental offices in California with nine or more employees.

Injury and Illness Prevention

California's Injury and Illness Prevention (IIP) program builds upon the federal OSHA mandates. Every employer in the state is required to establish, implement, and maintain an effective IIP program, which means you must:

- Identify the person responsible for the program's implementation
- Develop a system to ensure that employees comply with safe and healthy work practices
- Perform training, re-training, disciplinary actions, and any other measures deemed necessary to ensure compliance
- Establish a system for clearly communicating with employees about matters relating to occupational safety and health, including provisions to encourage employees to inform the employer of hazards at the work-site without fear of reprisal

Compliance with this provision requires meetings, training programs, postings (Box 8-3), written communication, a system of anonymous notification, labor-management safety and health committees, and any other means necessary to ensure proper communication.

Local Regulatory Compliance (San Francisco)

Business registration certificate

San Francisco requires dental practices to have a valid business registration certificate from the Office of the Treasurer and Tax Collector. A new

Box 8-3 **Examples of required postings in California dental offices**

- Notice to Employees of Disability Insurance
- Notice to Employees of Unemployment Insurance
- Notice to Employees of Paid Family Leave
- Notice to Employees of Pregnancy Leave
- Notice to Employees of Military Leave
- Notice to Employees of Workers' Compensation Carrier
- California and Federal Minimum Wage Notice
- Orders Regulating Wages, Hours and Working Conditions
- Pay Day Notice
- Equal Employment Opportunity Commission Nondiscrimination in Employment
- Nonharassment
- Time off to Vote
- Safety and Health Protection on the Job
- Emergency Action Plan
- Employee Polygraph Protection Act
- Whistleblowers Protection Act

practice must register for an initial certificate within 15 days of conducting business, at which time an annual fee is assessed. For new businesses, the first year's registration fee is based on the amount of tax due from its estimated annual payroll expenses, which is reported on the application for business registration. The registration and the annual fee are renewed at the beginning of the city's fiscal year (ie, July 1) and paid to the San Francisco Tax Collector.

Tax clearance

San Francisco requires a tax clearance when buying an existing practice even when no payment is exchanged in the transfer of ownership. A tax receipt from the Tax Collector will show that all of the seller's taxes on the practice are paid and no amount is due. In San Francisco, when a practice is sold, its business registration certificate is inactivated, which means that if a dentist buys a practice, he or she must submit a Request for Information Change to the Office of the Treasurer and Tax Collector.

Amalgam separator

The city and county of San Francisco mandate that each dental office must have an amalgam separator installed between the vacuum pump and the drain at its own expense. This is not optional. San Francisco maintains a list of preapproved amalgam separators, which are called *dental office pretreatment units*, with ISO 11143 specifications. The units must be replaced on a regular basis. Since the California Dental Association intervened, the exorbitant cost to purchase and install these units has markedly declined.

A wastewater discharge permit is issued by the San Francisco Public Utilities Commission after an office is inspected for amalgam separator installation and for compliance with the Dental Mercury Reduction Program. When a wastewater discharge permit is issued, a best management practices (BMPs) certification form is included. The signed certification form is submitted to the city to certify that the BMPs have been implemented.

Conclusion

Owning and operating a dental practice entails more than just clinical dentistry. As the manager of the business, the dentist is responsible to comply with multiple federal, state, and local regulations to protect patients, employees, and the environment. The state and local requirements described here related specifically to California and San Francisco, respectively. Whatever city and state in which you practice will have similar but distinct regulations, so it is important to do your research and make sure you are fully compliant to avoid potentially severe consequences.

Managing Managed Care

Michael Okuji, DDS, MPH, MBA

This chapter describes the managed care dental health system and how it impacts dental care delivery and payment in private practice. Managed care is different from indemnity insurance. Indemnity insurance focuses solely on payment for care, while managed care determines what kind of care is paid for and by whom it can be provided. Managed care payments account for a large share of all dental patient payments, which means that all dentists are economically and personally affected to some extent by the incursion of managed care.

The Evolution of Managed Care

Fifty years ago, the percentage of dental care expenditure in the United States covered by some form of third-party insurance was so small that it was reported to be zero.[1] Back then, 10% of the population utilized 67% of dental resources.[2]

From the 1960s to the 1980s, the nature of dental benefits was indemnity insurance, in which the insurance company indemnifies (ie, pays on behalf of) the beneficiary a portion of the dental care charge, while the patient pays the insurance deductible and copayment. The deductible is a specified amount a patient pays prior to the insurance company providing any payment. In some cases, like prophylaxis, the deductible is waived. The copayment is the amount the patient pays that is the difference between the insurance amount and the dentist's usual, customary, and reasonable fee (UCR). Typically the copayment is expressed as a

indemnity insurance
Insurance in which the insurance company indemnifies (ie, pays on behalf of) the beneficiary a portion of the medical charges, while the patient pays the insurance deductible and copayment.

deductible
A specified amount a patient pays prior to the insurance company providing any payment.

copayment
The amount the patient pays that is the difference between the insurance amount and the dentist's usual, customary, and reasonable fee (UCR).

percentage of UCR, like 20%. There was also an annual maximum (ie, cap) on how much the insurance company would pay. The only type of dental managed care program during this period was offered by the International Longshore and Warehouse Union health maintenance organization (HMO) dental plan through Dr Max Schoen's Southern California group dental practice.

When dentists join a PPO, they often avoid losing their existing patient base but still see a drop in revenue as a result of the discounted fees.

In the 1980s, preferred provider organizations (PPOs) began to emerge. A PPO is a type of managed care system similar to its HMO predecessor, but with larger provider networks (see chapter 5). The PPO contracts with dentists to become participating providers on a reduced fee-for-service basis with the promise of access to its beneficiaries. Many established dentists choose to become participating providers because they are fearful they will lose patients who can choose a participating provider for a guaranteed reduced fee. But, many dentists also find that they keep their existing patient base–but now at a lower fee. For a practice starting from scratch, the pro forma must account for the expected PPO discount. See chapters 7 and 10 for more detailed information.

Managed care systems control more than the costs of care—they also control how and by whom care is delivered.

For managed care systems, containing costs means more than just discounting fees. They institute preauthorization, appropriate and necessary treatment protocol, retrospective or concurrent review of treatment, and quality assurance programs that participating dentists agree to abide by. So while indemnity insurance is a system that finances services, managed care is a system that involves both the finance and delivery of dental care. The managed care company may fund and/or administer a plan, while third-party administrators and administrative services organizations manage and pay the claims on behalf of a self-insured group, employer, or plan.

A managed care company is licensed and regulated by the state in which it operates. Its mandate is to ensure that its beneficiaries have access to affordable care in facilities with providers that meet certain regulations and standards. For instance, a body of laws including statutes known as the Knox-Keene Health Care Service Plan Act covers California managed care plans. The California Department of Managed Health Care (DMHC) develops regulations to clarify the requirements of these statutes, overseeing some plans while the Department of Insurance oversees others. The DMHC designs and implements requirements for the financial benefit and health protection of the beneficiary, not the dentist.

To get an idea of the current magnitude of managed care penetration into dental care, consider that in 2007 the DMHC regulated 25 dental or dental/vision plans that enrolled 20 million (54%) of the state's total 37.7 million population[3,4] (Fig 9-1). Managed care payments now constitute a

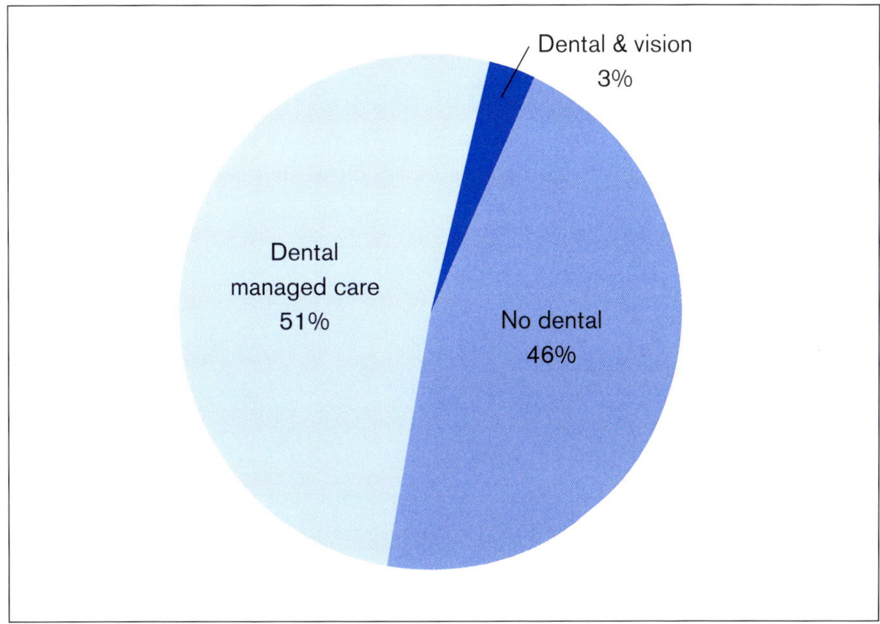

Fig 9-1 Patients enrolled in managed care dental plans in California in 2007. Data from the State of California.[3]

large portion of practice revenue, so much so that one-half of all dental revenue comes from direct managed care payments.[1] When the cash payments for deductibles and copayments from managed care patients are included, one could estimate that 70% of a practice's gross revenue comes from the managed care system. If that's true, is it really possible for dentists to financially survive outside of the managed care system?

Considering the extent of managed care's penetration into the dental health care system, it no longer seems feasible for dentists to financially survive outside of managed care plans.

Managed Care Programs

Managed care plans market a basket of programs, including PPOs, exclusive provider organizations (EPOs), and HMOs. Managed care plans may fund and administer these programs and provide their network of dentists, or for self-funding organizations like unions and large employers, they may provide only administrative services and their dentist network. Each of these programs is described below. To get a real-world view of managed care, talk with colleagues and fellow local dental society members about the different types of plans and working in the managed care system.

Preferred Provider Organizations (PPOs)

A PPO is a fee-for-service organization. A patient selects a participating provider dentist who agrees to charge a maximum or allowable fee. The plan's fee is published in a maximum or allowable fee schedule and is lower than the UCR fee. Fees for each discrete service rendered are submitted to the PPO for payment using the American Dental Association (ADA) Code on Dental Procedures and Nomenclature. The patient pays a deductible and copayment. Separate deductibles may apply for preventive, restorative, and "major" services.

Covered and noncovered services

Covered services are specified in the participating provider agreement, and only those services are paid by the plan. Not all services are covered, even if they're listed on the fee schedule. A covered service like prophylaxis may have no deductible and no copayment and may even have its reimbursement fee set at $0.

Some PPO plans may stipulate that a dentist has to limit the charge for a noncovered service to the plan's allowable fee.

A patient may elect to receive a noncovered service, and, in this situation, the dentist may be able to charge and collect the UCR fee from the patient. However, some plans may stipulate that a dentist has to limit the charge for a noncovered service to the plan's allowable listed fee.

Coverage outside of the PPO network

A patient enrolled in a PPO plan may seek care from a dentist outside of the network panel. This dentist is not restricted to the PPO fee; instead, the patient pays the out-of-network dentist the full difference between the PPO allowance and the dentist's UCR fee. In some instances, when a patient seeks care outside of the plan's panel of dentists, the plan sends payment to the patient, not to the dentist. However, since a managed care plan exists for the benefit of its enrollees, it's expected to exert leverage and direct enrollees to participating providers with whom they have contractual agreements, rather than providers outside of the network.

Participating provider agreement

To become a participating provider, a dentist must sign a provider agreement. Boxes 9-1 and 9-2 provide examples of the types of terms and inclusions that may be part of a provider agreement. Although a plan may offer many different managed care programs, a dentist does not need to participate in every program that the plan offers; instead, he or she can sign an agreement with one or more individual programs. A maximum

Box 9-1 Common contract terms in participating provider agreements

- Covered services
- Eligibility of beneficiary
- Compensation and remuneration
- Utilization review
- Quality assurance program
- Prior authorization
- Concurrent and retrospective review
- Term and length of agreement
- Termination
- Hold harmless–*Make sure a liability incurred as a result of a hold harmless provision in a contractual obligation is covered by your malpractice insurance.*
- Charge for noncovered service–*A plan may include a provision that stipulates the fee a dentist can charge for a noncovered service and/or a provision that precludes billing a patient for a noncovered service unless the patient is informed in writing of the noncovered service fee.*
- Appeal mechanism
- Dispute resolution
- Access to records
- Patient grievance procedures
- Coordination of benefits–*If the plan is secondary, does it pay the full difference between the primary amount and what the dentist charges? Does it pay its percentage of the difference between the primary amount and the dentist's charge (ie, a certain percentage of the balance), with the patient liable for some of the amount? Does it pay the difference between the primary amount and what the plan would have paid if it were primary?*
- Collection of the deductible and copayment–*A plan may specifically preclude the waiver of any deductible or copayment, reasoning that the waiver of part of a fee results in a lower fee, which should be the new UCR fee. A most-favored nations clause says a dentist will offer the plan the same discount he or she offers to any other plan.*
- Severability–*If one provision is held invalid, the remainder will be upheld.*
- Maximum or allowable fee schedule, or a protocol for obtaining one

fee schedule or table of allowances is attached to the agreement. For some plans this includes fees for noncovered procedures; however, if it does not, dentists can charge their UCR fee for a noncovered procedure. The agreement also lists certain administrative procedures, office protocols, and regulatory mandates by which the provider agrees to abide.

The agreement is a binding contract, so read and analyze it meticulously. Professional counsel is always recommended, either through an

Box 9-2 Common inclusions in participating provider agreements

- The company will establish and enforce policies and procedures to ensure compliance with state and federal regulations.
- The dentist agrees to complete treatment and cases in progress for a newly enrolled member.
- The dentist will continue to provide services for a certain period after termination from the plan.
- The dentist agrees to comply with company quality control and cost containment standards.
- The dentist allows the company access to dental records, books, and papers for the purposes of quality assessment, utilization, quality improvement, and investigation of a patient complaint.
- The dentist participates in audits and evaluations concurrently or retrospectively to establish necessity and appropriateness.
- In coordination of benefits, any excess payment exceeding the maximum plan fee is refunded to the plan.
- The plan is the sole source of payment, and any payment received from workers' compensation, auto, health, and casualty insurance is turned over to the company.
- The dentist holds harmless the company for any breach of the agreement, error, or omission.

attorney or the ADA and its state associations. The ADA offers a contract analysis program and a resource titled "What Every Dentist Should Know Before Signing a Dental Provider Contract," which is available to ADA members online. Your state dental association also should have an array of resources on managed care and provider agreements.

Exclusive Provider Organizations

In an EPO, the plan does not pay for any services provided by dentists outside of the network, which creates greater patient loyalty to provider dentists.

An EPO has the same features of a PPO except that dentists outside of the network panel are not paid for any dental services. A patient selecting a dentist outside the exclusive network panel pays for all dental care in full, which is a strong incentive for patients to select only participating provider dentists.

Health Maintenance Organizations

An HMO is a unique and different system. Unlike the PPO, it is not a fee-for-service plan. It doesn't reimburse a dentist for every discrete service;

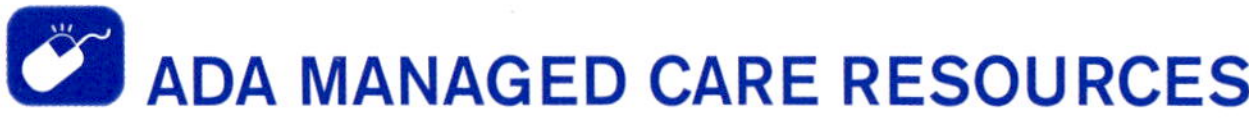

ADA MANAGED CARE RESOURCES

- www.ada.org/prof/resources/topics/managedcare

instead, the dentist is responsible for the comprehensive dental care of a specific number of patients for a specific time period.

An HMO plan is a capitation plan, which means that the plan pays the dentist a flat fee per member, per month (pmpm), which is paid whether or not a patient seeks dental care. For instance, a dentist with 100 patients with HMO coverage may be paid $25 pmpm (ie, $2,500 per month), whether or not a patient seeks care. Referrals are made to specialists contracted within the HMO.

In theory: *(1)* a dentist is assigned patients when a group signs up for the HMO, *(2)* the individual doesn't self-select an HMO because of preexisting conditions, *(3)* the group is stable with low employee turnover, *(4)* the group continues under this plan for a number of years, and *(5)* the dentist brings the group to a stable, healthy position where the patients remain in recall without further treatment for many years.

However, in reality, it's a poor plan that recruits a neglected patient group that easily switches plans, has high employee turnover, and assigns a new patient to a dentist only when he or she requests care, not when the patient first enrolls. Furthermore, for the HMO system to be successful, all of the players–the plan, the group, and the dentist–must share the same vision of dental care delivery. The HMO dentist assumes both the financial and dental care burden, and the financial risk is usually greater. To a much greater degree than a PPO dentist, the dentist in an HMO plan is required to have a thorough grounding in plan design, contracts, efficient delivery system, the economy of scale, and acute business acumen.

The reality of HMO plans rarely lives up to their theoretical potential, and HMO dentists take on a significant financial risk.

Case Example: Delta Dental Plan of California

Delta Dental Plan of California (Delta) is a Knox-Keene plan overseen by the DMHC. As stipulated in its participating dentist agreement, Delta conducts on-site quality assessment reviews of more than 1,000 offices annually as part of the Quality Assessment Program, which helps ensure that enrollees have access to appropriate, quality dental care that meets recognized practice standards.

Delta was conceived and has grown large in California, with enrollees equaling more than 44% of California's 37.7 million people.[3] Across the United States, Delta has more than 160,000 participating dentists, so the chance that you will become one of them is significant. Therefore, it is worthwhile for you to take the time to peruse the Delta website.

By definition, Delta is a managed care company. And, like many managed care companies, Delta offers a mix of plans.

- *Delta Dental Premier* is Delta's fee-for-service PPO network. The participating dentist agrees to adhere to Delta's policies, including the prohibition against billing a fee above the maximum for a service. There are deductibles and copayments, and, under the Delta Dental Premier table of allowances program, the plan pays a percentage of the allowance, but patients are responsible for the balance. Patients can elect to seek treatment from a nonparticipating dentist and pay the difference between Delta's payment and the dentist's UCR fee. Delta sends reimbursement checks directly to the patients who receive care from nonparticipating dentists.
- *Delta Dental PPO* is a different PPO plan that offers a deeper discount on fees than the premier plan with a smaller network of dentists. The participating dentist agrees to adhere to Delta's quality assessment, administrative, and other polices.
- *DeltaCare USA* is a prepaid HMO plan with no deductible. Dentists manage the comprehensive needs of the patient, including referrals to specialists, and receive a monthly capitation (pmpm) payment. This is not a fee-for-service plan, although it does have a copayment feature. Enrollees must select a primary care dentist from the DeltaCare USA network.
- *DentiCal* is California's Medicaid dental program that Delta administers through its DentiCal dentist network. Beneficiaries must visit a DentiCal network dentist, who is paid according to a fee schedule.
- *Healthy Families* is another California program administered by Delta Dental and three other dental plans to provide dental coverage to children of low-income working families. Most preventive, basic, and major restorative services are covered. Beneficiaries must select a network dentist, who is paid on a fee-for-service basis.
- *TRICARE Retiree Dental Program* is a dental benefit program for uniformed services retirees and their families that is administered by Delta Dental. This is a PPO program, so network dentists agree to accept the program's PPO fees. Direct payment is made only to Delta Dental dentists.
- *Delta Dental Patient Direct* is Delta's discounted fee-for-service dental plan for patients without dental benefits. Participating dentists agree to charge discounted fees to these patients and collect all of the fees directly from the patient. This is not an insurance plan.

Billing Issues

Cash flow is the key to the financial health of a dental practice, and, in an ideal dental world, the entire fee is collected when a service is rendered. However, in many locales, it's customary to bill the insurance company and collect only the deductible and estimated copayment from the patient at the time of service. (In the past, dentists would charge a fee for submitting a dental claim on behalf of a patient, but managed care companies explicitly prohibit this patient charge.) Other dentists collect the full fee up front and have the reimbursement check sent directly to the patient.

In the worst-case scenario, no payment is collected at the time of service, a claim is submitted to the insurance company, and payment is received in about 30 days. Then, the patient is billed the balance, which is hopefully paid in another 30 days. This means that nearly 60 days has passed since the original date of treatment with all of the attendant administrative costs before the procedure is paid in full–a cash-flow nightmare.

Electronic Claims Submission

To expedite managed care payments, dentists are turning to electronic claims submission (ECS), which most managed care companies accept, including Delta. An ECS is the quickest way to submit claims with attachments; an added benefit is that insurance payments can be electronically deposited into a bank account.

Electronic claims submission (ECS) is a relatively new but highly popular way for dentists to expedite managed care payments.

To use ECS, a computer that supports ECS software is required. The software will connect you to a dental claims clearinghouse, which transmits the ECS to the managed care company for a fee. You can get a clearinghouse referral from your software vendor, managed care company, or state dental association.

National Provider Identifier (NPI)

A national provider identifier (NPI) is required for dental claims submission, as well as access to ECS. As mentioned in chapter 8, an NPI is a unique numeric identifier that every health care provider uses for claim submission. It is part of the administrative simplification requirement established by the Health Insurance Portability and Accountability Act (HIPAA) to protect the security and privacy of health care information. It is required to submit a claim electronically, verify eligibility, or check a claim's status. Its purpose is to eliminate the need for different identifiers when sending electronic transactions. Having an NPI may eventually be required for all health care transactions, whether electronic or not. Remember that a single electronic transaction automatically puts you under the umbrella of HIPAA, so you'll be required to adhere to all HIPAA requirements and mandates for information protection and privacy. Be prepared for a steep HIPAA learning curve and compliance implementation.

A single electronic transaction automatically puts you under the umbrella of HIPAA, which means you'll be required to adhere to all HIPAA requirements and mandates for information protection and privacy.

Your NPI is permanent and won't change upon practice relocation. Having it doesn't require you to participate in any dental plan or to use electronic transactions, nor does it guarantee payment. It doesn't replace your social security number, state dental license number, Drug Enforcement Agency number, or your federal employer identification number.

Antitrust

Dentists rail against the perceived inequity of delivering expert dental care for a fee set by a managed care company. All they see is a large corporation wielding tremendous financial clout in the marketplace and arbitrarily setting low reimbursement rates to dentists. In their minds the countervailing force required to level the playing field is strength in numbers, to join other independent dentists to demand higher reimbursement or to leave the field altogether. They may imagine a group of dentists deciding to boycott the insurance companies as a veritable group of Davids defeating Goliath.

Resist the temptation to gather up like-minded dentists to discuss a reimbursement increase or a boycott of insurance companies. This is illegal anticompetitive price fixing, and the legal ramifications could be devastating.

Don't do it. Don't think it. Resist the temptation. It is illegal. An informal group of independent dentists who gather to discuss a reimbursement increase or a boycott are engaging in naked price fixing, which is a violation of the Sherman Antitrust Act. In fact, concerted action by even two independent dentists to restrain competition by raising prices is prohibited. Not fair to you, but true.

A group boycott by independent dentists to jointly raise reimbursement rates is always judged *per se* anticompetitive. Something that is illegal *per se* is an action that is inherently illegal regardless of the purpose, effect, or justification of the action based on relevant facts. This type of *per se* action, described as horizontal market arrangement among competitors, may amount to two sole proprietors meeting to grouse about a fee then jointly setting out to demand a fee increase. Even if two dentists jointly agree to *lower* their fee, that action may also be judged *per se* anticompetitive.

Antitrust action can be pursued as a civil or criminal action. A civil action is characterized by one private entity, such as an insurance company, suing another, such as a dentist. Private parties can bring suit for injuries stemming from antitrust actions. A criminal action is when the government files suit against an individual. Criminal antitrust penalties can range up to 10 years in jail and a $1 million fine, not to mention the excruciatingly high emotional and financial costs of a criminal defense.

Case Example: US v A. Lanoy Alston, DMD, PC

Let's look at one antitrust case involving a dentist. In a 1990 case, *US v A. Lanoy Alston, DMD, PC*, the government charged three Tucson dentists with engaging in a price-fixing conspiracy, which was the government's first criminal health care antitrust case against a health care practitioner in more than 50 years. The dentists allegedly met with 50 other local dentists at Dr Alston's Tucson dental office to discuss how copayments from an HMO plan had not risen for 10 years in Tucson, while copayments for the same services were raised during the same period in Phoenix. It's contended that Dr Alston, with encouragement from the local HMO representative, wrote a letter to the HMO asking them to raise the copayment and encouraged 50 local dentists to mail identical letters demanding a higher copayment as well. After the dentists mailed the identical letters, the HMO adopted the demanded fees.

A jury later convicted Dr Alston and two other defendants of antitrust violation. In January 1993, after appeals, the government reached a settlement whereby the charges were voluntarily dismissed, and Dr Alston pleaded *nolo contendere* (ie, no contest), was fined $5,000, was put on probation for 547 days, and was required to perform 250 hours of community service. Whew! Imagine 3 years of litigation on a criminal charge with endless hours of worry, countless hours in court, and an astronomical attorney's fee.

The short answer to how to avoid antitrust behavior is to never discuss fees with another independent dentist who is not affiliated with your practice. The long answer can be found on the ADA's website in the antitrust section, which has all the (albeit rather dry) information you need to get up to speed on the subject.

Never discuss fees with another independent dentist who is not affiliated with your practice.

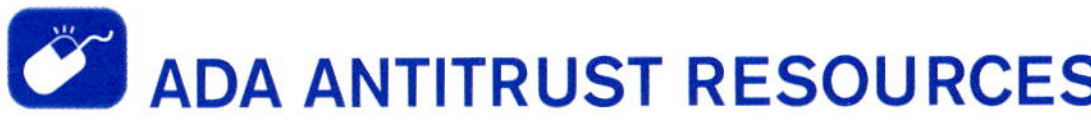

ADA ANTITRUST RESOURCES

- www.ada.org/prof/resources/topics/trust.asp

Conclusion

Managed care is here to stay. Its ubiquity in dental prepayment renders the traditional UCR system of pricing dental services all but archaic. The 21st century dentist is more challenged than dentists of any previous generation to deliver state-of-the-art dental care with high patient expectations in an economic climate of shrinking fees, exploding overhead, and unpredictable cash flow. It is highly important that you are prepared for the ramifications of the managed dental system in terms of treatment planning, record keeping, third-party oversight, and dental care delivery.

References

1. US Department of Health and Human Services, Centers for Medicare and Medicaid Services website. Historical National Health Expenditure Data [NHE web tables]. http://www.cms.hhs.gov/NationalHealthExpendData/downloads/tables.pdf. Accessed 30 December 2009.
2. Schoen MH. Observation of Selected Dental Services Under Two Prepayment Mechanisms [thesis]. Los Angeles: UCLA School of Public Health, 1969:13.
3. State of California, Department of Managed Health Care website. Complaint & arbitration decisions. 2007 independent medical review and complaint results. http://www.hmohelp.ca.gov/library/reports/complaint/2007.pdf. Accessed 30 December 2009.
4. Lawrence S. California population nears 38 million, LA tops 4 million. San Francisco Chronicle. May 1, 2007. http://www.sfgate.com/cgi-bin/article.cgi?f=/n/a/2007/05/01/state/n151653D18.DTL. Accessed 30 December 2009.

Designing a Business Plan

Scott Stafford, DDS, MBA
Frank Licari, DDS, MPH, MBA
Michael Okuji, DDS, MPH, MBA

A business plan should clearly describe your practice and the steps you'll take to manage its growth. It is the single most important document for your practice because, internally, it will guide your practice and, externally, it will be used to secure financing.

The business plan is used internally to forecast the needs of the practice and to monitor its progress. It's examined externally by banks and lending institutions to ascertain the credibility and the viability of the enterprise. Lenders rely heavily on this document in a startup practice because it's their sole source of information on which to judge the prospects of the practice.

While there is no universal template, your business plan should be no more than 30 pages. Use 24-lb, linen content, white or off-white paper. Format it with 1-inch margins, double-spaced lines, 12-point Times New Roman font, and include a header with your name, the date, and pagination.

A business plan can be written in many different ways, two of which are described in the sections that follow. Although an assertive, active voice is preferred over passive voice, there really is no best writing style. Two dentists may have wildly different takes on describing the same dental practice. The important factor of your business plan is to ensure that it precisely marks your path for you and your staff and clearly explains its vision, mission, and execution to a lender. See Appendix II for a sample business plan.

Business Plan 1

In dentistry, as in sports, we must prepare a game plan. A game plan shows a thorough study of the playing field and the development of a systematic approach to successfully playing the game. Having the desire to be successful is not enough. Entering to win is the culmination of a study of the numbers, evaluation of the demographics, sizing up of the competition, design of the operating budgets, and creation of the playbook: the business plan.

The business plan should cover, but not be limited to, the following items:

- Narrative
- Practice philosophy
- Consumer market analysis
- Demographic data and interpretation
- Timeline
- Marketing plan
- Goals
- Financial data

Narrative

The narrative is your chance to be heard and express your vision and your mission.

Simply put, the narrative is you telling your story. When the practice loan application goes before the bank committee and its underwriter, they don't know you and your passion for this project. The narrative is your chance to be heard and express your vision and your mission. The narrative explains how you see the practice and states the purpose of the dental business, how it functions, the environment in which it operates, and why the business will ultimately succeed.

Practice Philosophy

Your practice philosophy is how you approach the practice of dentistry, such as how you think patients should be treated. This section addresses the values and principles that guide you in developing your professional practice style. Also included in this section is how staff members will be recruited, trained, motivated, and maintained. This is important because the staff will convey your philosophy. They are in contact with patients as much as–if not more than–you will be and must promote your personal core values.

You can also use this section to draw from the good and not-so-good encounters you have already experienced that have helped develop your personal vision of how to treat patients who walk through the office door.

Consumer Market Analysis

A consumer market analysis is the area of the business plan that evaluates the environment in which the proposed practice is located. Even the best conceived practice struggles when it's placed in a market that is not compatible.

Even the best conceived practice struggles when it's placed in a market that is not compatible.

Not all seemingly attractive markets are appropriate for every type of dental practice. For example, there may be an area of Florida that is flourishing, where there is considerable new construction and an economic upswing. But what if the area's growth comes from a large influx of retiring baby boomers? That would make this a great opportunity for a prosthodontist, but not a pedodontist, whose practice may struggle or possibly fail.

Demographic data and interpretation

Age

Data on the median age of the occupants in the area are readily gathered and scrutinized. Are they older, younger, or right in the middle of the age spectrum? An older age group is beneficial to a prosthodontist or a general practice that offers advanced restorative and implant-based dentistry. The younger age group is perfect for a pediatric, orthodontic, or general practice that caters to young patients, while the middle age group is well suited for the general dentist and the advanced restorative dentist.

Families

Demographic reports will show the average family size in the area. With a larger median family size, you can get more bang for your buck in marketing efforts. If demographics show a median family size of five members, including three children, the practice gains five new patients by just winning Mom. If the demographics reveal a median two-member family household with husband and wife and no children, then the marketing effort gain is only two new patients per household.

Owners versus renters

Another important demographic report is determining what percentage of the local population owns versus rents its residence. Owners reward a single marketing effort with a potential patient for many years into the future. Renters are more transient, and a single marketing effort may bring a patient for only 1 to 2 years, after which a new marketing effort is required to acquire the new renter who took over the apartment after the first renter moved out.

Education level

People who attain higher levels of education place a greater emphasis on health care than the general population, so the number of people who hold advanced degrees is a demographic worth investigating. They also tend to have higher incomes, which allow for more discretionary dental care expenditures.

Household income

As with many other statistics, you can compare the local income figures to the state or national averages to determine whether the area of interest is above or below the state or national average household income. This can help determine if the area selected has the economic resources to access the dental services you intend to deliver.

Timeline

Your timeline should show the exact timing and sequence of events in the startup of the dental practice. As with anything important, planning is everything, and the steps to take when starting a business are best not left to chance. The startup timeline can take anywhere from a matter of months to a matter of years depending on the location, existing condition of the facility, amount of construction required, availability of contractors, and employee market. Box 10-1 shows a sample 12-month startup timeline.

Marketing Plan

A marketing plan shows how you plan to promote your practice in parallel with your practice philosophy and mission. It is divided into external and internal marketing plans.

External marketing

External marketing is directed toward the population that you want to attract to your practice. The message or theme should be in line with your

Box 10-1 Sample 12-month startup timeline

12 months:	Select location.
	Finalize facility design.
11 months:	Final selection of building contractor.
	Finalize lease with leasing agent.
10 months:	Finalize bank funding.
9 months:	Receive bids from dental suppliers for equipment.
8 months:	Develop relationships with insurance broker, certified public accountant, and lawyer.
7 months:	Obtain building permits.
6 months:	Write staff manual and job descriptions.
5 months:	Establish relationship with dental suppliers.
4 months:	Order dental supplies.
	Begin staff recruitment.
3 months:	Apply for state, local, and professional licenses.
	Apply to state for incorporation.
2 months:	Finalize staff selection.
	Finalize bank financing.
1 month:	Establish dental laboratory relationships.
	Finalize construction.
	Finalize equipment placement and installation.
0 months:	Open the door.

philosophy so that you don't attract patients who want services or features that you don't offer. External marketing efforts should be monitored using a concrete marker of success–return on investment (ROI). A marketing effort that delivers \$3 in dental treatment for every \$1 of expenditure would have an excellent ROI ratio of 3:1. As you can already imagine, this requires keeping meticulous records of expenditure in each marketing effort and tracking, from patient feedback, which marketing avenue brought patients to your office. Some examples of external marketing are:

External marketing conveys the philosophy and features of your practice to the specific patient population that you want to attract to your practice.

- Direct mailing
- Classified advertising
- Billboards
- Bus benches
- External office signage

Internal marketing

The goal of internal marketing is to inspire loyalty in current patients.

Internal marketing is directed toward current patients and is intended to reinforce a patient's decision to continue visiting your practice. Some examples of internal marketing efforts include:

- Offering refreshments in the reception area
- Contacting patients after a procedure to follow up
- Sending birthday cards to patients
- Sponsoring patients in civic events

Goals

Success is what you strive for in dental practice, but what does practice success mean to you? It might be a practice that grows at a rate of 25% per year. Or maybe it is one that supports two full-time doctors or produces enough income to allow you to retire in 20 years.

Once you have determined how you define practice success, you must begin to set goals that will measure your progress toward that success. These practice goals should be realistic, quantifiable achievements that you can work toward. It is easy to say, "I want a million-dollar practice," and just sit back and wait for the money to roll in–but it won't happen. A million-dollar practice is an attainable goal, but this system for achieving it will clearly fail. An effective goal system must have:

Goals are most effective when you make them quantifiable, monitor them at an appropriate frequency, and use the data they provide to adjust performance and improve outcome.

- A clear, well-stated description of the goal to be achieved
- A concrete plan to achieve the goal
- A time frame allotted to achieve the goal
- Planned intervals to check and monitor the progress toward the goal

Box 10-2 gives an example of an effective goal system. The sample goal was chosen for a couple of reasons. First, it does not deal with money. So often we think that all practice goals must involve money, eg, how much money can be produced or collected, how much money is produced through hygiene services, or how much money can be saved by reducing overhead. Although these are important considerations, they should not define your practice, nor should they be your only indicators of success. You should have some goals that are quantifiable, yet not completely monetarily based.

Second, this goal allows you to address several key questions about how you are running your practice, such as:

Box 10-2 Example of an effective goal system

- *Goal:* A 95% acceptance rate of treatment plans proposed to patients.
- *Plan:* Provide a comprehensive, well-thought-out treatment plan with the input and preferences of the patient acknowledged. Communicate the need for, benefits of, and risks of not following the plan to the patient, and provide financial options to aid the patient in pursuing the treatment plan.
- *Time frame:* Measure success at 6 months.
- *Intervals:* Once a month, compare the number of treatment plans proposed with the number accepted. Evaluate and compare the accepted and unaccepted treatment plans. Assess whether all the steps of the plan were followed for the treatment plans that weren't accepted, then make modifications in the treatment plan and presentation as needed to increase acceptance rate.

- Do you communicate well with patients?
- Do you meet your patients' needs?
- Do you provide financial options so patients can pursue their dental needs?
- Do you learn from your successes and failures by monitoring results?

Another important point to remember as you set goals for your practice is that it is easy to confuse a professional goal with a personal goal. If the practice prospers, then so do you. If you personally prosper, then often the practice does as well, but your success in life is not strictly dependent on the success of the dental practice. Try to develop a separate set of practice goals and personal goals. The practice is an organization with many factors and participants, and it is important to involve your staff and patients in achieving the practice goals. With personal goals, however, the attainment is pretty much up to you.

Goals make us stretch and reach for new levels of accomplishments just beyond our grasp. Be reasonable when setting what you want to achieve. If after a period of time you and your team don't reach a goal, readjust how you pursue it. Consult with a colleague, a mentor, or a consultant for more tools to achieve what you want. Don't become discouraged if you have difficulty achieving a particular goal; instead, become inventive and inspire your dental team.

Estimated Production and Collection

A Month	B Number of patient visits	C Average fee per patient visit	D Current month production (B × C)	E Production collected at time of service	F Current month production collected (D × E)
1st	40	$170	$6,800	49%	$3,332
2nd	50	$170	$8,500	52%	$4,420
3rd	60	$185	$11,100	58%	$6,438
4th	70	$185	$12,950	54%	$6,993
5th	90	$185	$16,650	58%	$9,657
6th	125	$150	$18,750	53%	$9,938
7th	125	$150	$18,750	51%	$9,563
8th	130	$175	$22,750	55%	$12,513
9th	135	$175	$23,625	51%	$12,049
10th	135	$180	$24,300	51%	$12,393
11th	140	$180	$25,200	52%	$13,104
12th	160	$200	$32,000	56%	$17,920
Total	**1,260**		**$221,375**		**$118,318**

Notes:

B Number of patient visits, not number of total patients
C Average fee charged per patient; factor in managed care contracts
D Monthly production; multiply patient visits by average fee per visit (B × C)
E Percent of production expected to be collected at the time of service
F Total dollars collected from current month's production (D × E)
G Total dollars earned but not collected this month; may include insurance due (D – F)
H Total dollars paid on account from previous months' treatment (insurance, payment plans, etc)
I Total dollars owed you by paients (previous month's I + G – H)
J Total dollars collected this month (F + H)

Fig 10-1 Spreadsheet for estimating first year's production and collection.

Financial Data

Although it is not necessary to prepare a multitude of financial spreadsheets, you do need to show potential lending institutions how you anticipate money to flow through the dental practice and, ultimately, how you plan to pay them back.

Many books on business plan development advise the reader to prepare countless pages of financial spreadsheets. Although such an excessive number of reports is unnecessary, it is important to provide potential lending institutions information on how you anticipate money to flow through the dental practice and, ultimately, how you plan to pay them back. For a new practice startup these data are at best educated guesses; however, in the case of a practice purchase the previous owner can provide historical data for the practice.

G Current month production receivable (D – F)	H Received on account	I Total accounts receivable (previous I + G – H)	J Current total collections (F + H)
$3,468	$0	$3,468	$3,332
$4,080	$3,383	$4,165	$7,803
$4,662	$4,229	$4,598	$10,667
$5,957	$5,522	$5,033	$12,515
$6,993	$6,443	$5,583	$16,100
$8,813	$8,283	$6,113	$18,221
$9,188	$9,328	$5,972	$18,891
$10,238	$9,328	$6,882	$21,841
$11,576	$11,318	$7,140	$23,367
$11,907	$11,753	$7,294	$24,146
$12,096	$12,089	$7,301	$25,193
$14,080	$12,537	$8,844	$30,457
	$94,213	**$8,844**	**$212,531**

Production and collection

Estimated production and collection figures are broken down on a monthly basis, which is the easiest way to monitor financial progress through the first year of practice. Fig 10-1 shows a basic spreadsheet that will help you perform the computations that will determine the level of expected production and collection on a monthly, quarterly, and annual basis. This particular example is for a startup practice.

The number of patient visits (column B) starts low (approximately two per day) then grows at a fairly rapid pace. In the purchase of an existing practice, the patient-visit numbers start higher but grow at a slower rate.

		Pro Forma Cash Flow				
		Month 1	Month 2	Month 3	Month 4	Month 5
1	Production	$6,800	$8,500	$11,100	$12,950	$16,650
2	Collection	$5,440	$7,803	$10,667	$12,515	$16,100
3	Practice Expenses					
a	Staff salary	$4,320	$4,320	$4,320	$4,320	$4,320
b	Rent/mortgage	$2,800	$2,800	$2,800	$2,800	$2,800
c	Utilites including telephone	$650	$650	$650	$650	$650
d	Office supplies	$136	$170	$222	$259	$333
e	Dental supplies	$408	$510	$666	$777	$999
f	Taxes (including payroll)	$431	$431	$431	$432	$432
g	Dues, licenses, subscriptions	$75	$75	$75	$75	$75
h	Insurance	$280	$280	$280	$280	$280
i	Professional fees (CPA, attorney, etc.)	$200	$200	$200	$200	$200
j	Laboratory fees	$680	$850	$1,110	$1,295	$1,665
k	Meetings and CE	$20	$20	$30	$50	$50
l	Marketing	$680	$850	$1,110	$1,295	$1,665
4	Total Practice Expenses	$10,680	$11,156	$11,894	$12,433	$13,469
5	Profit (Loss)	($5,240)	($3,353)	($1,227)	$82	$2,631
6	Less:					
a	Dentist's salary	$5,000	$5,000	$5,000	$5,000	$5,000
b	Bank loan	$1,608	$1,608	$1,608	$1,608	$1,608
7	Cash Surplus (Deficit)	($11,848)	($9,961)	($7,835)	($6,526)	($3,977)
8	Cumulative		($21,809)	($29,644)	($36,170)	($40,147)

Fig 10-2 Pro forma cash flow statement.

Estimate the average fee per visit (column C) to start the cash flow calculations for the practice (column D), then, based on your practice philosophy and vision, determine how much of the money is collected at the time of service (column E). If you have a strictly fee-for-service practice without insurance, there may be a 100% collection at the time of service, but if the practice accepts assignment of dental insurance benefits, then the collection at the time of service is between 50% and 80%. Another factor that practice philosophy influences is the financial policy. A practice that diligently pursues the collection of outstanding debt should collect money owed fairly quickly and in full, which positively impacts the received on account figures (column H) on the spreadsheet.

Forecasted financial data must be backed up by firm practice philosophy guidelines and financial policies.

All of these numbers are very important for the practice, but, without practice philosophy guidelines and firm financial policies, the economic success of the practice is still left to chance.

Month 6	Month 7	Month 8	Month 9	Month 10	Month 11	Month 12	Year-to-Date
$18,750	$18,750	$22,750	$23,625	$24,300	$25,200	$32,000	$221,375
$18,221	$18,891	$21,841	$23,367	$24,146	$25,193	$30,457	$214,641
$7,145	$7,145	$7,145	$7,145	$7,145	$7,145	$7,145	$71,615
$2,800	$2,800	$2,800	$2,800	$2,800	$2,800	$2,800	$33,600
$650	$650	$650	$650	$650	$650	$650	$7,800
$375	$375	$455	$473	$486	$504	$640	$4,428
$1,125	$1,125	$1,365	$1,418	$1,458	$1,512	$1,920	$13,283
$715	$715	$715	$715	$715	$715	$715	$7,162
$75	$75	$75	$75	$75	$75	$75	$900
$280	$280	$280	$280	$280	$280	$280	$3,360
$200	$200	$200	$200	$200	$200	$200	$2,400
$1,875	$1,875	$2,275	$2,363	$2,430	$2,520	$3,200	$22,138
$50	$100	$100	$100	$100	$100	$100	$820
$1,875	$938	$1,138	$1,181	$1,215	$1,260	$1,600	$14,807
$17,165	**$16,278**	**$17,198**	**$17,400**	**$17,554**	**$17,761**	**$19,325**	**$182,313**
$1,056	$2,613	$4,643	$5,967	$6,592	$7,432	$11,132	$32,328
$5,000	$5,000	$6,000	$6,000	$6,000	$6,000	$6,000	$65,000
$1,608	$1,608	$1,608	$1,608	$1,608	$1,608	$1,608	$19,296
($5,552)	($3,995)	($2,965)	($1,641)	($1,016)	($176)	$3,524	($51,968)
($45,699)	($49,694)	($52,659)	($54,300)	($55,316)	($55,492)	($51,968)	

First-year cash flow

The next step is to estimate the expenses of the practice and how they relate to the practice operations. Figure 10-2 is a pro forma cash flow statement that lists the expenses that the practice incurred to carry out production and collection each month. Rows 1 and 2 show figures generated from Fig 10-1. The expenses the practice has incurred for each month are subtracted from the monthly collection amount.

One way to determine how much to estimate for each expense category is to look at industry benchmarks (Table 10-1). However, in the infancy stage of the practice the percentages are always higher than the benchmarks because they are a function of production. The production level is low early in a practice because you are just starting out, and the practice is building. Like the production and collection figures, the expenses you estimate will be a reflection of your practice philosophy.

The expenses you estimate will be a reflection of your practice philosophy and financial policies.

Table 10-1 Important historical benchmarks for a general dental practice*

Expense category	Percentage of production
Staff	23.0–28.0
Tax including payroll	10.0
Laboratory fees	10.0
Dental supplies	6.0
Rent	3.0
Marketing	0.5–1.5
Information technology	1.0–3.0

*These are historical guidelines for a general dental practice to keep overhead between 55% to 65%. Information technology is a growing part of new practices and may begin to represent a greater expense category.

Staff salary

The number of assistants you feel the practice needs is directly reflected in the labor costs incurred. In addition, the level of expertise you are looking for in employees affects the amount you will pay to hire and retain them. You could, for example, at the start of your practice hire two assistants, one with a few years of experience and the other with very little experience, in the anticipation that the veteran will train the novice. This way you avoid incurring the expense of two expert assistants, yet you still have an experienced staff member who won't require training.

Whether you or a hygienist performs prophylaxis and periodontal treatment also can directly affect labor costs and possibly production values. While avoiding the cost of paying a hygienist may seem like a cost savings, if you perform so many hygiene functions that restorative appointments are limited, then the productive potential of the practice is limited. A good compromise is to perform your own hygiene procedures in the beginning, when the practice is slow, then hire a hygienist when the practice becomes busy. In this way, you limit early labor costs, then add staff to increase production when the practice is ready.

It is often prudent to limit early labor costs by hiring minimal staff; however, be sure to increase staff as production picks up to avoid limiting the growth of your practice.

Office facility

The facility you select should be in harmony with your practice philosophy but never a huge financial burden to the practice. While you would not locate a pediatric practice in a warehouse district just because the space is cheap, you must also weigh the expense of a very upscale, high-rent setting with the expected return. This is where a practice philosophy can help clarify your decision. It states whom you want to serve and how you want to serve them. By determining the clientele that you want to target, you'll better define where to find them and how to offer services to meet their needs.

Although space for function, growth, and expansion with qualified staff are required even at low production levels, too much additional expense overwhelms cash flow. An example of this is in rent or lease cost. Rent is usually targeted to be approximately 3% of production, but in a startup practice, this ratio is initially much higher because office space is rented to allow for growth even in the absence of a steady patient stream. The question is, how much growth in how much time is anticipated? Most leases are from 5 to 10 years, which is a manageable time period for making growth assumptions. In other words, even though you will potentially practice for 25 years or more, you don't need to anticipate the growth of the practice for your whole career–just the duration of the lease.

For example, a confident solo general dentist will anticipate needing a dental hygienist within a fairly short time frame, and therefore may choose an office with four treatment rooms at the beginning of the practice. The dentist will operate in two rooms, while the hygienist operates in one room with an additional room for emergencies. An option is to design and equip only three of the rooms until the practice needs the fourth room. This way, the initial cost to equip the facility is lessened until the practice production meets the need for the additional room. Again, always minimize the expense the practice must pay until production warrants the expansion of the facility and staff.

It is a good idea to keep facility and equipment costs at a minimum until increased production warrants expanding your capacity.

Fixed, variable, and semivariable expenses

Other office expenses are described as fixed, variable, and semivariable. An example of a fixed expense is the monthly rent. Rent does not change, no matter the amount of treatment produced, money collected, or patients seen. An example of a variable expense is a laboratory fee. The more patients treated in a month, the higher the monthly laboratory expense, and, conversely, the fewer patients treated, the lower the laboratory expense will be in a month. An example of a semivariable expense is labor cost. Monthly labor cost is fairy stable, but if there are days the office is closed, the labor cost may go down, and if extra hours in a day or an extra day is required to service patients, the employees work extra hours, and labor costs go up. The goal is to maximize revenue generated from your fixed costs while limiting increases in your variable expenses.

fixed expense
An expense that remains the same regardless of production.

variable expense
An expense that changes in direct relationship to production.

semivariable expense
An expense that is relatively stable, but influenced by either exaggerated highs or lows in production.

Below-the-line expenses

After all of the general office expenses are tallied on the spreadsheet, there are two last payments to make: one to the bank, and one to the boss (lines 6a and 6b in Fig 10-2). These two expenses are known as *below-the-line expenses* because they are subtracted from the net office profit (loss) line (line 5 in Fig 10-2), which is also called the *bottom line*. Although the daily expense of running the practice is important, the bank note and the owner salary are equally essential and must be satisfied on a monthly basis.

The bank note is determined by the amount of money borrowed to purchase or start the practice and the terms of the note (interest rate and payback period). This bank note payment is determined by performing an amortization calculation (see chapter 7), which determines the monthly payment divided into principal and interest for the time period needed to pay the money back. The average time most lending institutions allow a dentist to repay a loan is 84 months (7 years). Some banks allow 1-year, interest-only payments and then 7 years of principal and interest payments. You might consider the interest-only option only for a startup that is tight on cash, but never on the purchase of an existing practice unless the facility needs major updating. The money requested in the loan package for a startup will include funds to purchase equipment, initial supplies, office furnishings and fixtures, leasehold improvements, and working capital. Working capital is an important factor that is discussed later in the next section.

When creating a personal budget, keep in mind that expenses drastically increase once you leave dental school.

The second below-the-line expense is the owner's salary, which is determined by forecasting a personal budget. If you are like many dental students and recent graduates, you may think you won't need much money to live on, but the reality is that expenses drastically increase once you leave dental school. The roommate who shared your rent and food expenses moves out after graduation. You won't have any paid medical, disability, life, or malpractice insurance, all of which may be required by a lender before you can purchase a practice. Perhaps the biggest expense looming in the not-so-distant future is the student loan payment, since forbearance usually expires 6 months after graduation. Given the current rate of dental student indebtedness, the monthly loan payment consumes quite a large portion of the personal budget. Add up these examples of personal expenses–not to mention other personal wants, such as a new home or car–to create your personal budget and determine your salary.

Working capital

Once you determine how much money is collected in a month, subtract the operating expense, the bank note, and the owner's salary. The resulting number determines whether the practice turned a profit or took a loss for the month (line 7 in Fig 10-2). There is usually no profit in the first month of a new startup practice; to be even more realistic, there is usually no profit for the first 6 to 10 months. In Fig 10-2, line 7 is a negative number until the 12th month, which means that this is that point at which the practice and personal enterprise have stopped losing money.

It simply takes more capital to start up or to purchase a dental practice than can be made in the first few months. Given this fact, you must borrow working capital, which is extra funds borrowed from the bank to get by until the practice turns a profit. Working capital is calculated to meet the practice shortfall (loss) after factoring in personal need in addition to the hard assets and leasehold improvements. It is sometimes paid out in a lump sum, but more often it is offered as a line of credit.

working capital
Extra funds borrowed from the bank to run the practice until it turns a profit.

If the money is disbursed as a lump sum, interest is immediately charged and accrued on the entire amount. However, if the money is disbursed as a line of credit, interest is charged and accrued on just the amount taken and only as you use the money. The amount of working capital needed is–at best–an educated guess. But, given historical practice startup numbers and the dental industry norms, working capital needs can be estimated fairly close to the actual need. It makes sense to request a few percent more in the working capital budget than you've initially calculated for several reasons. First, it's not an exact science and you can't foresee everything that might happen in your first year of practice. Second, it is better if down the road you have to tell the bank that you do not need that last $10,000 after all, rather than that you need an additional $10,000.

To be safe, request a few percent more than your estimate for the working capital budget.

Each time money is taken out of the line of credit to pay for the practice or for a personal expense, the total loan amount goes up, the amortization table is recalculated, and the monthly loan payment increases. The best way to project working capital need is to run several months of projections and keep a running total of accumulated cash surplus or shortfall, as shown in line 8 of Fig 10-2. The highest amount of cumulative cash deficit ($55,492 in the 11th month in Fig 10-2) represents approximately how much working capital you should request in the business plan. It's important to note, again, that this is not an exact science, so you may want to ask for more funds to allow for a margin of safety.

This may appear to be a considerable amount of money to borrow in addition to all the equipment costs and the money spent to get the space ready for a dental office, but be advised that the number one reason for dental practice failure is undercapitalization, which means that the practice doesn't have enough money to meet current expenses. All kinds of

undercapitalization
Situation in which the practice doesn't have enough money to meet current expenses.

business owners–not just dental practice owners–often think that they should operate on a shoestring budget, but then they can't satisfy all the financial obligations in the early years of the business. Consequently, they fail and go out of business because they didn't budget enough working capital for the times when the business encountered a cash flow crisis.

Reducing the loan amount

If the size of the entire loan package is unwieldy and uncomfortable, then certain measures can be taken to reduce the initial loan amount. Bear in mind that deep cutbacks may impede the practice's ability to offer core services that go hand-in-hand with the practice's vision and mission. It would be analogous to a McDonald's restaurant that decides to cut expenses by discontinuing its drive-thru service. How much of its sales would be lost due to its inability to deliver fast food to its customers in their cars?

As mentioned previously, one fairly safe and effective way a dental office can save money is to scale back on capacity. Perhaps only three dental treatment rooms are initially equipped in an office designed and finished for four treatment rooms. While the compressor, vacuum system, and other fixed essentials are already in place, the cost of the additional chair, task light, unit, cabinetry, and other pieces of equipment is saved until production (and need) is ramped up. The absolute minimally required computer stations for a startup can be purchased, with more stations purchased later as they are required. Maybe a part-time hygienist is initially hired to contain costs, and the dentist performs some of the hygiene functions until a full schedule of patients is attained.

Don't skimp on what is truly necessary to achieve the quality core services inherent to your vision.

Bear in mind that skimping on certain areas isn't advised because the practice suffers when these areas are underfunded. Areas that fit in this category include external and internal marketing, use of a reputable dental laboratory, and using high-quality dental supplies. Oftentimes when a fledgling practice uses a cut-rate dental laboratory or cheap supplies, the treatment outcomes become unpredictable or unreliable. Retreatment and refabrication are expensive and result in bad patient relations, so strike a balance between what is truly necessary to achieve the quality core services inherent to your vision and the costs associated with these expenditures.

Business Plan 2

A meaningful business plan requires thorough research and meticulous attention to detail. Remember that it's the game plan to start a practice. Think through each step as if your money is at risk–because it is. And, speaking of risk, don't be afraid to take calculated leaps of faith. Business decisions are about taking action in the face of incomplete knowledge and uncertainty. That's the nature of business in general and dental practice in particular.

The business plan should begin with a clear statement of your vision and mission, which comprises the internal compass that guides you through a career. The rest of the business plan presents the steps you will take to implement that vision. Develop a concise, meaningful, and personal point of view and then promulgate it. The qualitative description of the business, environment, process, and quantitative pro forma expectations flow naturally from your vision and mission, reflecting your style and worldview. You will make decisions about starting a new practice versus purchasing an existing practice; leasing versus buying space; urban versus suburban; risky versus safe; and exuberant versus staid. Plan every step in advance.

Your writing style should be personal, and the content should include these key elements:

- Cover sheet
- Executive summary
- Table of contents
- Mission and vision statements
- The practice
- The market
- Competition
- Marketing
- The management team
- Cash need
- Pro forma financial statements
- Appendix

Cover Sheet

A cover sheet includes your full name, your local mailing address, email address, and local telephone number. Use a telephone number at which you can easily be reached, like a cellular phone number. Don't list a temporary address or the proposed office address; rather, list the address where documents will be mailed. You'll want to make sure you are easily accessible.

Executive Summary

The executive summary, also known as the *statement of purpose*, summarizes the proposed practice and capital (ie, money) needed. It should be clear, concise, and limited to a single page. Use this section to make a good first impression.

Table of Contents

Including a table of contents with page references makes it easy for the reader to access information in your business plan proposal. Do not place supporting information here; the appropriate place for this documentation, which includes the dental license, lease agreement, architectural design, equipment inventory, and anything that supports the main body, is the appendix at the end of the business plan.

Mission and Vision Statements

Imagine what your dental practice will be like 10 years from now. As you look into the future, carefully reflect on all aspects of this practice. Is it the type of practice that you want? Are you enjoying practicing dentistry? Does your practice provide you with the income level and financial security that you expect? Do you like its location? Do you think that you have the right people working for you? Are your patients satisfied with the services that are provided by your office?

Placing yourself on the direct path to achieve the practice you want means taking the time to develop the type of mission and vision statements that will guide your practice to success.

In 10 years your practice will be *exactly* how you designed it, whether you planned it like that or not because successes–and, for that matter, failures–do not happen by accident. They are planned events that develop over time. Placing yourself on the direct path to achieve the practice you want means taking the time to develop the type of mission and vision statements that will guide your practice to success.

Mission statement

It probably seems obvious that mission statements are appropriate for large corporations such as Home Depot, Holiday Inn, Microsoft, or

United Airlines. In these large corporations it would be impossible to get all employees to move in the right direction if there wasn't an overarching mission statement to guide them. Think of how different the culture is among the employees of a Holiday Inn versus those of a Ritz-Carlton. Both groups of employees work within the hotel industry, yet they serve very different missions. Holiday Inn employees focus on offering "today's business and leisure travelers dependability, friendly service, and modern attractive facilities at excellent value,"[1] whereas Ritz-Carlton employees pledge "to provide the finest personal service and facilities for our guests who will always enjoy a warm, relaxed, yet refined ambience."[2] The behavior and actions of employees in each of these organizations are therefore very different and yet successful for the customers that they are trying to serve.

In your own dental practice you have the opportunity to treat patients in the particular way in which you feel they should be treated. For example, do you think that all emergencies should be seen immediately? Do you emphasize esthetics? Is prevention the cornerstone of your practice? Is restoring your patients back to oral health your main objective? Do you feel that your patients deserve a spa treatment as they come to your practice for care? Each option offers its own unique circumstances for creating the type of practice that you desire. Consider, however, that there is also the potential that multiple points of focus may be in conflict with each other. For example, providing a spa experience for your patients may not allow you the time or proper environment for treating all emergency patients immediately.

It is important that the specific nuances unique to your style of treating patients are fully communicated to your staff. If you do not have a clearly defined mission, your office staff will develop their own mission based on their own values and their day-to-day routine in the practice. This type of unstated mission can become deeply ingrained in the culture of your practice and almost impossible to change. Therefore, communicating your practice's mission to your employees is vital to having the kind of practice you desire. Whether your employees have been there for a long time or have just been hired, your ability to direct their actions toward your mission will predict your overall success, which means that you need to take your time to develop a well thought-out mission statement.

Communicating your practice's mission to your employees is vital to having the kind of practice you desire.

Developing the mission statement

Developing a mission statement is not as easy as it may sound. It requires thought and honest reflection on what values are most important to you and which ones you want to emphasize. A good way to approach this process is to think of yourself as a patient who is entering your practice for the first time. Now think about what elements would be the most important in making this experience with a new dentist a good one. Would it be:

- How far in advance you had to schedule the appointment
- How easy the office is to locate or access
- Whether and how you are greeted
- How comfortable the waiting room is
- How long you wait in the waiting area
- The ambience of the office
- The dentist's attitude and approach
- Your satisfaction with the treatment
- Whether the dentist answered your questions
- Whether someone explained the total cost of treatment
- Accurate and efficient billing

Take time to develop a list of any additional factors that you feel are important to a positive patient experience. Begin to define and describe in greater detail how you would like the process to go. This will help you begin to establish areas that are important to you as you develop your unique style of practicing dentistry. It is also a good idea to find out what areas of practice are important to members of your staff.

At this point you should be ready to draft your mission statement. Box 10-3 shows some examples of mission statements. Solicit feedback from your staff members once you have drafted your mission statement. Take the time to listen to their input. It is important that your staff members believe in the mission statement as much as you do and that they buy into its implementation. Once your mission statement is finalized, actively communicate it to your patients and referral sources. A framed copy should be in your waiting room and in a prominent place in your office for your staff to see every day. Also make sure to post it on your website.

Vision statement

Once you have a mission statement, develop a vision statement or action plan. In the hectic pace of working in a dental office it is sometimes easy to lose sight of where you would like to be in the future. Think of your vision statement as a time-directed road map to your goals. Unlike the mission statement, which is a public document communicated to patients

Box 10-3 Sample mission statements

- Our mission is to provide the highest quality dental care to all of our patients. We are committed to working with our patients to develop healthy smiles that can last a lifetime.
- Our mission is to develop a professional relationship with all of our patients, founded on a commitment to provide them with the best possible patient care and personal service.
- We are dedicated to providing dental care to patients in a relaxing and welcoming atmosphere. Your total experience is important to us, and we will strive to make you as comfortable as possible.
- Our mission is to make ourselves available whenever you need us. We provide convenient hours for working individuals and 24-hour emergency coverage.
- We are committed to providing patients with a lifetime of oral health by emphasizing preventive dental care.

and staff, the vision statement is an internal document only meant to be shared between you and your staff. The vision statement should look into the future and consider where you would like to be 3, 5, or maybe 10 years from now. Would you like to own more than one office? Do you want to be the office providing the most cosmetic dentistry or implant procedures in your city, your county, or your state?

Developing the vision statement

The vision statement requires that you look introspectively into what you really want professionally and personally, so take some time to reflect on where your career has taken you and dream of where you want to be in the future. This is your opportunity to develop your vision and create goals that may challenge you to acquire new skills and reach into some untapped resources. For example, if you want to own more than one office in 5 years, you may have to develop skills in office design, construction, real estate, or business plan development. As you open this second office you may have to delegate parts of the project to an office manager or associate and develop more of your leadership and management skills. Setting forth on this path through a clear vision statement will be the catalyst that initiates the change. Most people think about how nice it would be to have a second office but rarely get past this first phase. Successful people develop a clear vision of what they want to achieve, then use their vision to systematically set the goals needed for its success. Box 10-4 presents sample vision statements.

Successful people develop a clear vision of what they want to achieve, then use their vision to systematically set the goals needed for its success.

Box 10-4 Sample vision statements

- Our dental practice will be the first choice of patients in this area who desire cosmetic dental services by 2015.
- Our dental practice will provide dental services to patients throughout the entire county from two locations by 2013.
- Over the next 4 years we will successfully transform our general dental practice into an oral health care spa while retaining 90% of our current patients.

Once you've clearly defined your mission and vision statements, you are ready to write a business plan that fits your goals, addresses your strengths, suits your personality, and guides you through the game. But don't let it stop there. Keep a copy of your vision statement in your office and review it every 2 to 3 years to assess your progress and adjust as needed.

The Practice

This section of the business plan describes the physical location, office, and dental services that the practice will provide. Describe the city and neighborhood, the building and population served, and the particulars of the office space itself. When describing the dental services offered, make sure to describe the skills and means available to effectively deliver the service.

The office lease is a key item described in this section, but the lease documents themselves should go in the appendix. A lease has an initial term and option(s) to renew (eg, entering into a 5-year lease with two additional 5-year options to renew at a stated renewal rate). The monthly lease payment is fixed for the initial term with an escalation clause for subsequent options. The ability to sublet (ie, allow another dentist to practice in the office) or assign the lease (ie, allow another dentist to assume the lease) is negotiable. The leased square footage in a multitenant building is the actual useable space or includes a "load" factor, which is the proportionate share of common space (eg, a hallway or restroom). The responsibility to pay for utilities and janitorial service, including medical and biohazardous waste disposal, is negotiable, but more often included in the lease for modern high-rise buildings than for small or single-tenant buildings.

In a gross lease, the tenant pays a fixed amount while the owner pays for all of the expenses to operate the property such as insurance, property tax, and maintenance. If you sign a single-net lease, this means that the tenant pays the proportionate property tax, while a double-net lease means that the tenant pays the proportionate property tax as well as property insurance. In addition, there is also a triple-net lease, which means that the tenant pays the proportionate property tax, property insurance, and maintenance costs. A single-tenant property is usually leased as a triple-net.

gross lease
Arrangement in which the tenant pays a fixed amount while the owner pays for all of the expenses to operate the property, such as insurance, property tax, and maintenance.

single-net lease
The tenant pays a fixed amount plus the proportionate property tax; the owner covers insurance and maintenance.

double-net lease
The tenant pays a fixed amount plus the proportionate property tax and insurance; the owner pays for maintenance.

triple-net lease
The tenant pays a fixed amount as well as the proportionate property tax, insurance, and maintenance costs.

Office buildout, leasehold improvement, or tenant improvement is the amount the owner agrees to pay to bring the property up to your specifications to do business. It is paid to offset contractor fees or as a monthly lease reduction for a specified amount of time. Except for minor cosmetic changes, improvements to a property require a local building permit, and issues such as copper versus plastic plumbing and the storage and venting of large G- or H-size nitrous oxide tanks fall under local ordinance. Improvements must be in compliance with public accommodation mandates of the Americans with Disabilities Act, such as entrance ramps, width of hallways, bathroom accessibility, and doorknob design.

The Market

The market is the local environment, including demographic, economic, and other population elements that impact access to dental care. The purpose of this section is to pinpoint the target patient population.

Demographics

Demographics are important because they illuminate the nature of a practice location in terms of the socioeconomic condition and transience of the surrounding population. To be useful, demographic information should focus on the relevant referral radius. In urban areas it's measured in city blocks or even can be limited to a single high-rise building, like One Embarcadero Center in San Francisco, where you can find all the patients needed to fill a practice. In the suburbs, the relevant referral radius is usually the local school district, while in rural areas it is measured in counties.

Demographic information should be analyzed in terms of how patients usually access care. Do they seek care near their home or their office?

Demographic analysis should also consider the commuting patterns of workers into, out of, and through the practice area. How many people commute into a neighboring financial district or out of a nearby residential area? In addition, the demographics should reveal the population's dental sophistication and their source of dental payment. Do they have the type of insurance and disposable income to pay for all dental services, including advanced, sophisticated care? Is the prototypical dental patient in the target population a young professional with robust dental insurance and little previous treatment, like a Silicon Valley computer programmer? Is it a soccer mom with young children and a working spouse? Is it a financial executive with ample insurance but scant time for oral health care? Or is it a senior with chronic health and dental issues with limited financial resources for health care except for Medicare?

Competition

Competition describes the other dentists in your market area. What services do they offer? How do they attract patients? Are there idiosyncratic barriers to entering into this market? The best place to start this research is through the American Dental Association's online member directory. It lists dentists by state, city, year of graduation, specialty, dental school, whether the listing is a home or office address, and principal occupation (eg, "private practice for more than 30 hours a week" or "dental school faculty"). The year of graduation gives you insight into where competitors are in terms of their career curve. Are they startups like you or in the growth, maturity, or decline stages? The local business phone directory can also give the flavor of the dental community. What features are emphasized in the practices' names and advertisements? Do they compete on convenient hours, low price, dental plans accepted, cosmetic service, or sedation and comfort?

Marketing

Marketing is how you intend to attract patients and defines how you propose to compete. You can market yourself (ie, advertise) in external and internal ways.

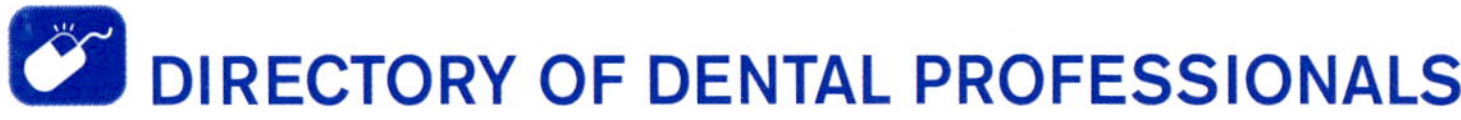

DIRECTORY OF DENTAL PROFESSIONALS

- American Dental Association: www.ada.org/members/directory/index.asp

External method

External marketing methods are those that reach out to new people whom you want to attract to your office. It focuses on reach and depth. The reach is the amount of people you want to market to: the entire city, the financial district, the school district, or one office high-rise? Depth refers to how often and in how many ways you want to market to these people: one mass mailing, one newspaper advertisement, repeated flyers, or expert speaker engagements? Reaching out without depth is ineffectual.

reach
The amount of people targeted in a marketing effort.

depth
How often and in how many ways a marketing effort accesses a target audience.

External marketing can be as simple as walking into neighborhood businesses to let them know you're accepting new patients and leave a business card or poster. It can be talking to the Parent Teacher Association about silver amalgam fillings or to the rotary club about the connection between periodontal disease and cardiovascular disease or volunteering for the local health fair.

External advertising can also consist of office signage, billboards, a mailed brochure, or a website. Be sure to mention any unique or attractive features of your practice, such as Saturday office hours, available nitrous oxide, or a staff member who speaks Russian.

Internal method

Internal marketing encompasses the efforts you make to retain patients by meeting their needs and wants. These efforts result in satisfaction that they convey to family, friends, and coworkers who become potential new patients. Internal marketing may be the range of services offered, the skill with which care is delivered, and the attention to patient satisfaction. Maybe it's price, location, or office hours. Internal marketing can include digital printouts of radiographs with notations, digital before and after photographs, or a brochure on how removable braces work. Although that nifty toothbrush kit in a bag with your name is a nice touch, the most effective internal advertising method is still the word-of-mouth personal referral of a satisfied patient.

The most effective internal advertising method is still the word-of-mouth personal referral of a satisfied patient.

The Management Team

Include your resume, which should be no longer than one page, in the Management Team section. Highlight any relevant training and experience. Describe how your education, training, and experience prepare you to deliver the proposed dental care and manage and market the practice. List key professional advisers, including your accountant, attorney, architect, designer, equipment specialist, and consultants, as well as the unique qualities they possess for the team. Are they familiar with dentists and dental practice? Have they worked with dental startups? Identify the internal staff members and their responsibilities and background, then describe the timeline in which they will join the team and how that will enhance the delivery of care.

Cash Need

Purchase only what you need, and make sure each purchase has a tangible source of repayment.

The section on cash need describes how money will be spent in the practice. The buildout requirement, equipment, supply, furnishing, and fixture costs are written as a line-item list. It's natural to dream about top-of-the-line, cutting edge pieces of equipment placed in an architectural digest setting, but this is the time for a big dose of reality. The business plan should balance the practice needs and wants. Each purchase must have a tangible source of repayment. Purchase and use exactly what you need and nothing more. Consider equipping only the first operatory initially, then the second operatory in 9 months. Wait to purchase the in-office dental ceramic milling machine until the laboratory bill exceeds $75,000 a year. Nothing cripples an enterprise faster than an equipment loan that can't be serviced with the current cash flow.

Similarly, a large inventory of supplies ties up cash that is sorely needed elsewhere. Do you really need all those implant parts when you are treating just one case a month? Try to formulate a just-in-time, first-in, first-out (FIFO) supply system to avoid the out-of-date, stale inventory that a last-in, first-out (LIFO) system creates. A FIFO just-in-time inventory system is most feasible when combined with reliable courier delivery.

The full amount of cash need is the first-year working capital shortfall (ie, the combined practice and personal shortfall), as determined by the pro forma cash flow, which is provided as supporting documentation in the next section. As the pro forma cash flow will show, working capital need isn't spread equally throughout the year, nor is it linear. Shortfall occurs and randomly spikes throughout the year. Although working capital can be rolled into the initial practice loan, a separate line of credit is preferred. As explained in chapter 7, a line of credit is a source of funds in a preapproved amount that can be accessed by writing a check when needed. It has an annual fee to maintain the account at a fixed or variable rate, and it is a revolving line of credit (ie, cash can be borrowed again once it has been repaid into the account). New owners usually seek the largest line of credit available since cash flow is precarious in the first year of a new practice and interest is charged only on the amount used.

New owners usually seek the largest line of credit available since cash flow is precarious in the first year of a new practice and interest is charged only on the amount used.

Pro Forma Financial Statements

Pro forma financial statements are generated using the expected future financial performance of a business based on its historical past performance or the past performance of similar businesses, including expected revenue, expenses, income, asset acquisition, and cash flow. Although an existing practice has historical financial data, there is a degree of uncertainty regarding whether they accurately predict expected returns. Therefore, it is important to analyze the quality of the data. Are the revenue, expenses, and assets directly attributable to business operation, or are they superfluous, tangential personal items? Is the general trend upward, level, or downward curving? In short, can past performance predict future production?

There are no historical data in a startup practice, so comparable financial data from neighboring practices must be used, but only with caution. Determine what items are directly comparable with a startup business and what is idiosyncratic to an ongoing enterprise. Consider such things as whether the source of revenue is managed care as well as the number and wage level of staff members. The ultimate goal of the pro forma is to reflect the best-guess expected financial outcome as accurately as possible within the framework of uncertainty.

The ultimate goal of the pro forma is to reflect the best-guess expected financial outcome as accurately as possible within the framework of uncertainty.

Two pro forma statements that should be included in your business plan are the balance sheet and the cash flow statement. They should include information for both the dental practice and your personal account.

Balance sheet

The balance sheet states the net worth of the practice at one point in time and includes your dental degree, an intangible key asset often overlooked. This intangible asset is the basis for future income production and is analogous to goodwill on the balance sheet. See chapter 7 for more information.

Cash flow statement

A pro forma cash flow statement is more appropriate for determining cash need for the dental practice business plan than an income statement. The traditional income statement includes a line for depreciation, a non-cash item. Adding depreciation distorts the real month-to-month cash need projection. What you really want to calculate is the real cash-in income and cash-out expense transactions that lead to operating income or loss in the dental practice. This means that you do want to include the business loan payment–even though it is a financing issue, not an operating one–because it is a cash-out event that influences cash need.

Personal Annual Expense Sheet

Personal Year 1	**Annual**	**Month**	**Quarter**	**Semiannual**
Rent	24,000	2,000	–	–
Utilities	1,200	100	–	–
Food	6,000	500	–	–
Entertainment	2,400	200	–	–
Clothes	2,000	–	500	–
Personal	1,200	100	–	–
Automobile	4,800	400	–	–
Automobile-gas	1,200	100	–	–
Insurance-auto	800	–	–	400
Insurance-health	3,000	–	750	–
Insurance-disability	2,000	–	–	1,000
Insurance-life	1,500	–	–	750
Medical expense	1,000	–	250	–
Subtotal	51,100	3,400	1,500	2,150
Student loan payment	17,805	1,484		
125,000	–			
120 months	–			
7.50%	–			
Total	**68,905**	**4,884**	**1,500**	**2,150**

Fig 10-3 Personal annual expense sheet.

What is left is a modified cash flow statement that resembles a checkbook register. It shows cash-in revenue as checks and credit card deposits into a checking account and cash-out expenses as checks written to pay expenses such as wages and supplies. Accounts receivable and accounts payable are not considered here because they are not cash-in-hand items. The pro forma cash flow statement covers a specific accounting period on a month-to-month basis. The example provided here covers a 12-month period; however, a 24-month period is preferable for a startup practice. In addition, for internal analysis, it is a good idea to prepare separate statements based on both best- and worst-case scenarios.

Preparing a pro forma cash flow statement

You don't need specialized business plan software to prepare your pro forma cash flow statement; a customized statement can be easily prepared for the specific needs of a dental practice in a spreadsheet program like Microsoft Excel. In separate worksheets in one workbook file, create per-

Practice Annual Expense Sheet

Business Year 1	Annual	Month	Quarter	Semiannual
Salaries-staff	75,000	6,250	–	–
Payroll taxes	7,000	–	1,750	–
Benefits	4,000	–	1,000	–
Salaries-hygienist	–	–	–	–
Rent	30,960	2,580	–	–
Advertising and promotion	12,000	1,000	–	–
Stationery and supply	2,000	–	500	–
Computer and software	3,000	–	750	–
Insurance	4,000	–	1,000	–
Legal and accounting	2,000	–	500	–
Miscellaneous	2,400	200	–	–
Telephone	3,000	250	–	–
Dues and subscription	2,500	–	–	1,250
Laundry	1,200	100	–	–
Repair and maintanence	1,500	125	–	–
Licenses	1,500	–	–	750
Taxes	1,000	–	–	500
Utilities	1,200	100	–	–
Other	–	–	–	–
Other	–	–	–	–
Other	–	–	–	–
Other	–	–	–	–
Laboratory (10 months)	20,000	2,000	–	–
Dental supplies	5,000	–	1,250	–
Continuing education	1,200	–	300	–
Janitorial	1,200	100	–	–
Other	–	–	–	–
Other	–	–	–	–
Other	–	–	–	–
Other	–	–	–	–
Business loan payment	42,733	3,561	–	–
300,000	–	–	–	–
120 months	–	–	–	–
7.50%	–	–	–	–
	–	–	–	–
Total annual	**224,393**	**16,266**	**7,050**	**2,500**

Fig 10-4 Practice annual expense sheet.

sonal and practice annual expense sheets (Figs 10-3 and 10-4) as well as a personal cash flow statement (Fig 10-5). Using the figures from these sheets, create your final combined personal and practice cash flow state-

Personal Pro Forma Cash Flow Statement

CASH IN	Month 1	Month 2	Month 3	Month 4	Month 5
WAGES					
W-2 Job 1	7,000	6,000	5,000	4,000	3,000
W-2 Job 2	3,000	2,000	1,000	1,000	1,000
Total wages	10,000	8,000	6,000	5,000	4,000
CASH OUT					
PERSONAL EXPENSE					
Rent	2,000	2,000	2,000	2,000	2,000
Utilities	100	100	100	100	100
Food	500	500	500	500	500
Entertainment	200	200	200	200	200
Clothes	-	-	500	-	-
Personal	100	100	100	100	100
Automobile	400	400	400	400	400
Automobile-gas	100	100	100	100	100
Insurance-auto	-	400	-	-	-
Insurance-health	750	-	-	750	-
Insurance-disability	-	-	-	-	-
Insurance-life	-	-	750	-	-
Medical	-	-	-	-	250
Subtotal personal expense	4,150	3,800	4,650	4,150	3,650
Student loan	1,484	1,484	1,484	1,484	1,484
Total personal expense	5,634	5,284	6,134	5,634	5,134
NET PERSONAL INCOME (LOSS)	4,366	2,716	(134)	(634)	(1,134)

Fig 10-5 Personal pro forma cash flow statement.

ment (Fig 10-6) in the same workbook. This allows data to be easily linked between the worksheets.

Revenue Revenue is money collected for services rendered. In the first months expect little revenue generation; in fact, you may wait up to 45 days to collect money for billed services. The "Returns and allowances" line is where bad debt or uncollectible debt is recorded. When calculating revenue, keep in mind that it is never linear. Don't expect or forecast

Month 6	Month 7	Month 8	Month 9	Month 10	Month 11	Month 12	YTD
2,000	1,000	-	-	-	-	-	28,000
1,000	1,000	1,000	-	-	-	-	11,000
3,000	2,000	1,000	-	-	-	-	39,000
2,000	2,000	2,000	2,000	2,000	2,000	2,000	24,000
100	100	100	100	100	100	100	1,200
500	500	500	500	500	500	500	6,000
200	200	200	200	200	200	200	2,400
500	-	-	500	-	-	500	2,000
100	100	100	100	100	100	100	1,200
400	400	400	400	400	400	400	4,800
100	100	100	100	100	100	100	1,200
-	-	400	-	-	-	-	800
-	750	-	-	-	750	-	3,000
1,000	-	-	-	-	1,000	-	2,000
-	-	750	-	-	-	-	1,500
-	250	-	-	250	-	250	1,000
4,900	4,400	4,550	3,900	3,650	5,150	4,150	51,100
1,484	1,484	1,484	1,484	1,484	1,484	1,484	17,805
6,384	5,884	6,034	5,384	5,134	6,634	5,634	68,905
(3,384)	(3,884)	(5,034)	(5,384)	(5,134)	(6,634)	(5,634)	(29,905)

the revenue line to go up every month; there are months when revenue steeply declines.

Expenses Expenses are linked from your practice expense sheet (see Fig 10-4). They are allocated by category then ranked from highest dollar amount to lowest. Make each category meaningful. For instance, separate employees into different categories such as "staff" and "hygienist" to track the impact of a change in hours or wages to the bottom line. Also

Practice and Personal Pro Forma Cash Flow Statement

CASH IN	Month 1	Month 2	Month 3	Month 4	Month 5
REVENUE					
Dental revenue	5,000	7,500	10,000	12,500	15,000
Returns and allowances	-	-	-	-	-
Total revenue	5,000	7,500	10,000	12,500	15,000
CASH OUT					
FIXED EXPENSE					
Salaries-staff	3,250	3,250	3,250	3,250	6,250
Payroll taxes	-	-	875	-	-
Benefits	-	-	-	-	-
Salaries-hygienist	-	-	-	-	-
Rent	2,580	2,580	2,580	2,580	2,580
Advertising and promotion	1,000	1,000	1,000	1,000	1,000
Stationery and supply	-	-	-	500	-
Computer and software	-	750	-	-	750
Insurance	1,000	-	-	1,000	-
Legal and accounting	-	-	500	-	-
Miscellaneous	200	200	200	200	200
Telephone	250	250	250	250	250
Dues and subscription	-	-	1,250	-	-
Laundry	100	100	100	100	100
Repair and maintanence	125	125	125	125	125
Licenses	-	-	-	-	-
Taxes	-	-	-	-	-
Utilities	100	100	100	100	100
Other	-	-	-	-	-
Other	-	-	-	-	-
Total fixed expense	8,605	8,355	10,230	9,105	11,355
VARIABLE EXPENSE					
Laboratory	-	500	750	1,000	1,500
Dental supplies	-	-	-	-	-
Continuing education	-	-	-	-	-
Janitorial	100	100	100	100	100
Other	-	-	-	-	-
Other	-	-	-	-	-
Total variable expense	100	600	850	1,100	1,600
Total operating expense	8,705	8,955	11,080	10,205	12,955
Operating income (loss)	(3,705)	(1,455)	(1,080)	2,295	2,045
LOAN PAYMENT					
Line of credit	-	-	-	-	-
Business loan	-	-	-	3,561	3,561
Total loan payments	-	-	-	3,561	3,561
Net income (loss)	(3,705)	(1,455)	(1,080)	(1,266)	(1,516)
PERSONAL INCOME (LOSS)	4,366	2,716	(134)	(634)	(1,134)
Total monthly cash surplus (need)	661	1,261	(1,214)	(1,900)	(2,650)

Fig 10-6 Practice and personal pro forma cash flow statement.

Month 6	Month 7	Month 8	Month 9	Month 10	Month 11	Month 12	YTD
10,000	15,000	17,500	20,000	22,500	25,000	27,500	187,500
-	-	-	-	-	-	-	-
10,000	15,000	17,500	20,000	22,500	25,000	27,500	187,500
6,250	6,250	6,250	6,250	6,250	6,250	6,250	63,000
875	-	-	1,750	-	-	1,750	5,250
-	-	-	1,000	-	-	1,000	2,000
-	-	-	-	-	-	-	-
2,580	2,580	2,580	2,580	2,580	2,580	2,580	30,960
1,000	1,000	1,000	1,000	1,000	1,000	1,000	12,000
-	500	-	-	500	-	500	2,000
-	-	750	-	-	750	-	3,000
-	1,000	-	-	1,000	-	-	4,000
500	-	-	500	-	-	500	2,000
200	200	200	200	200	200	200	2,400
250	250	250	250	250	250	250	3,000
-	-	-	1,250	-	-	-	2,500
100	100	100	100	100	100	100	1,200
125	125	125	125	125	125	125	1,500
750	-	-	-	-	-	750	1,500
-	500	-	-	-	-	500	1,000
100	100	100	100	100	100	100	1,200
-	-	-	-	-	-	-	-
-	-	-	-	-	-	-	-
12,730	12,605	11,355	15,105	12,105	11,355	15,605	138,510
2,000	2,000	2,000	2,000	2,000	2,000	2,000	17,750
1,250	-	-	-	1,250	-	-	2,500
-	-	-	-	-	-	-	-
100	100	100	100	100	100	100	1,200
-	-	-	-	-	-	-	-
-	-	-	-	-	-	-	-
3,350	2,100	2,100	2,100	3,350	2,100	2,100	21,450
16,080	14,705	13,455	17,205	15,455	13,455	17,705	159,960
(6,080)	295	4,045	2,795	7,045	11,545	9,795	27,540
-	-	-	-	-	-	-	-
3,561	3,561	3,561	3,561	3,561	3,561	3,561	32,049
3,561	3,561	3,561	3,561	3,561	3,561	3,561	32,049
(9,641)	(3,266)	484	(766)	3,484	7,984	6,234	(4,509)
(3,384)	(3,884)	(5,034)	(5,384)	(5,134)	(6,634)	(5,634)	(29,905)
(13,025)	(7,150)	(4,550)	(6,150)	(1,650)	1,350	600	(34,415)

be sure to allocate each expense category appropriately over the 12-month period. Some expenses are spread evenly over monthly, quarterly, or semiannual payments, eg, payroll tax is paid quarterly, while insurance, tax, license, dues, and subscriptions are paid either quarterly or semiannually. For a new practice, keep in mind that laboratory, dental supplies, and office expenses lag by approximately 60 to 90 days. In such cases, even though an expense may be incurred in month 1, you should not forecast it as an expense until you would actually pay it (eg, month 3).

Most expenses are fixed, which means that the expense isn't dependent on the number of patients treated and can incur at any level of output, including zero, while a variable expense occurs only when a patient is treated. Of course, even fixed expenses are variable over the long run: rent is renegotiated, employees are hired or fired, wages are raised or lowered, and assets are bought or sold. Laboratory expense and dental supplies are two important variable expenses.

Expense categories are totaled to arrive at a total operating expense, also referred to as *expense before interest, tax, depreciation, and amortization (EBITDA)*, which is then subtracted from the operating revenue to arrive at an operating income or loss (see Fig 10-6; also see chapter 7).

Loan payment The loan payment is entered on the next line. The loan payment is a cash-out event and important to determining your cash need. Most financial institutions offer a grace period of up to 6 months with no payments or interest-only payments, so you can omit a loan payment for the first few months. You can use one of the many loan calculators available on the Internet to estimate the amortized monthly payment for your practice loan (see also chapter 7).

Subtract the practice loan payment from the operational income or loss to arrive at net income or loss. This is your bottom line, which represents either a positive or negative cash flow. It is volatile and will fluctuate wildly during the first 12 to 24 months (Fig 10-7).

Personal income (loss) Now, add the personal income or loss from the personal pro forma cash flow statement (see Fig 10-5) to arrive at the total cash surplus or need per month for the 12-month period (see Fig 10-6). Remember that total cash need is forecasted monthly because practice net income (loss) varies greatly on a monthly basis (see Fig 10-7).

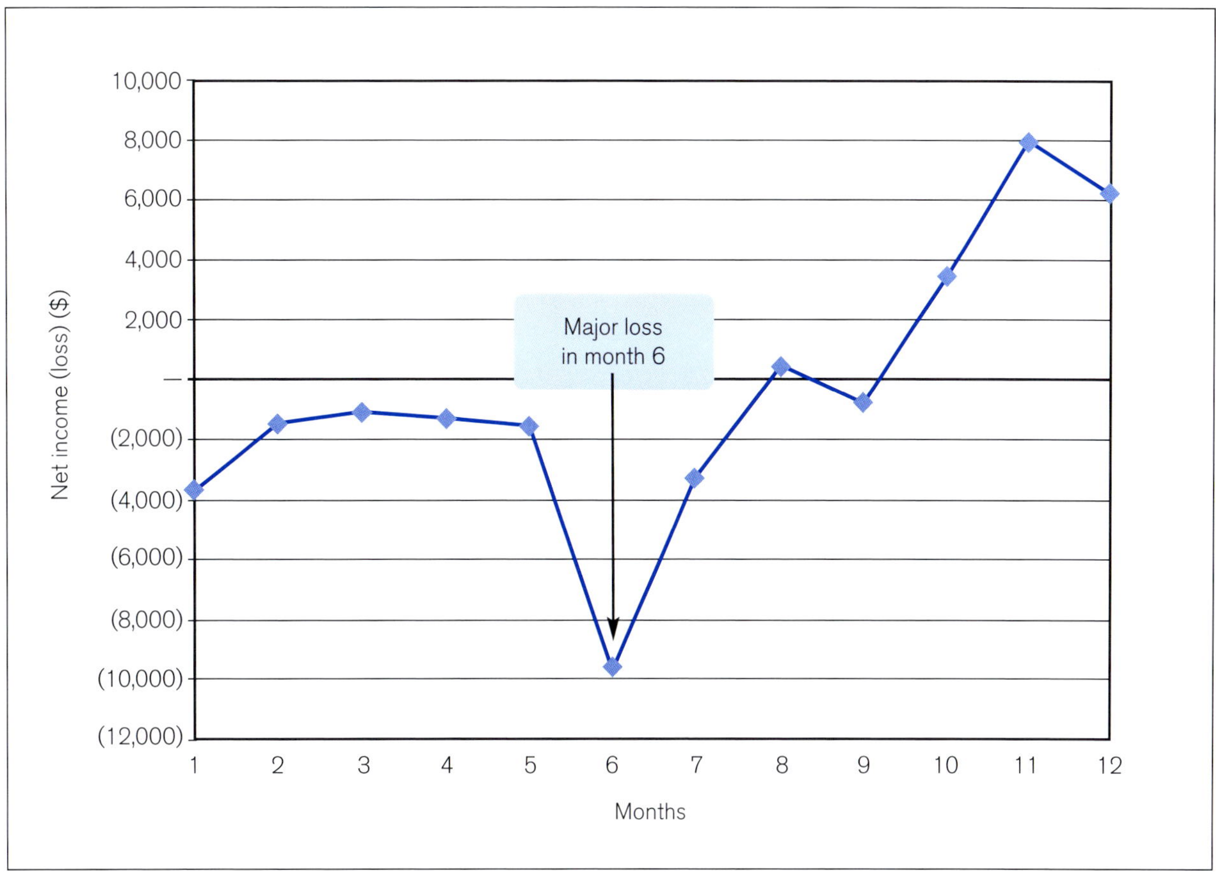

Fig 10-7 Fluctuations in monthly practice net income (loss).

Appendix

Any additional supporting documentation should be included in the appendix. These documents include anything that can be used as a basis for projections or lend gravitas to the business plan.

Some of these documents include:

- Resume
- Dental license
- Drug Enforcement Administration license
- Credit report and FICO score
- Personal income tax return
- Personal debt
- Office lease

- Equipment and supply
- Furniture and fixture
- Contractor estimate
- Office blueprint
- Area map of local businesses
- Area map of local dentists
- Website sample

Conclusion

When learning to play a game, there are two different concepts that must be understood: *(1)* how to play the game, which includes basic information about goals, limits, and how to score, and *(2)* the strategies and tactics of the game, ie, the plays you run or moves you execute. These business plans represent two individual strategies for playing the same game. As you write your own business plan, remember that everyone is bound by the same set of rules when playing the game, but it is those who best execute their strategies and tactics who win.

References

1. Holiday Inn website. Holiday Inn Fact Sheet. Updated November 10, 2009. http://www.ihgplc.com/files/pdf/factsheets/factsheet_holidayinn.pdf. Accessed 28 December 2009.
2. The Ritz-Carlton Hotel Company. Gold standards: The credo. http://corporate.ritzcarlton.com/en/About/GoldStandards.htm. Accessed 10 August 2009.

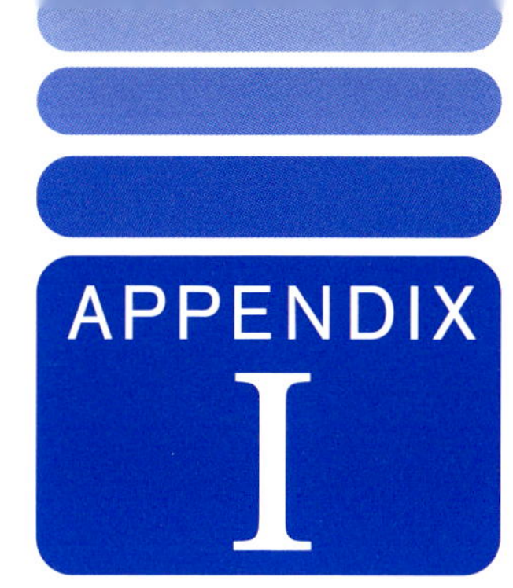

Valuation of Two Dental Practices

David Okuji, DDS, MBA

Let's run a valuation exercise to bracket the price ranges of two hypothetical dental practices using three methods to evaluate and determine acceptable ranges of purchase price: the market sales, capitalized earnings, and investment yield approaches.[1] Data for the two hypothetical practices are presented in Table I-1. Assume that the loan terms require 100% financing at an 8.0% fixed annual interest rate with a 15-year term.

Market Sales Approach

The market sales approach utilizes historical sales information to determine the value of a practice. Historically, dental practices sell for between 50% and 100% of their annual net revenue (Table I-2), a price that includes tangible and intangible (ie, goodwill) assets. This approach gives a broad view of the seller's asking price compared with most dental practices. It usually places the asking price on the high end of the market.

Table I-1 Two hypothetical practices (annualized data)

	Practice 1	Practice 2
Asking price	$1 million	$400,000
Revenue	$1 million	$400,000
Operating expense	$500,000	$200,000
Operating overhead	50%	50%
Operating income (ie, cash flow to buyer)	$500,000	$200,000
Loan payment	$114,678	$45,871
Pretax income after loan payment	$385,322	$154,129

Table I-2 Market sales approach to valuation of hypothetical practices

Annual revenue estimator (%)	Practice 1 value ($)	Practice 2 value ($)
100	1 million	400,000
90	900,000	360,000
80	800,000	320,000
70	700,000	280,000
60	600,000	240,000
50	500,000	200,000

Capitalized Earnings Approach

The capitalized earnings approach assumes that value is related to financial risk and reward, such that:

$$\text{Fair market value} = \frac{\text{Annual net return}}{\text{Capitalization rate}}$$

Annual Net Return

Annual net return is ascertained as if the buyer is a passive investor in the practice opportunity and the annual net return equals the annual net operating income (less a reasonable compensation paid to another dentist to

Table I-3 Capitalized earnings approach to valuation of hypothetical practices

Factor	Practice 1	Practice 2
Annual operating income	$500,000	$200,000
Less dentist compensation	$120,000	$120,000
Annual return	$380,000	$80,000
Capitalization rate	25.51%	25.51%
Market value	$1,489,612	$313,603
Asking price	$1,000,000	$400,000
Market value as % of asking price	149%	78%

provide dental services). For this example, we will assume that the other dentist is hired for $600 per day for 200 days per year for an annual compensation of $120,000.

Capitalization Rate

The capitalization rate is determined by:

- The sum of the average market return at valuation date
- Risk premium for business size
- Risk specific to the business

We will use a capitalization rate of 25.51% to find the market value of our hypothetical practices (Table I-3). The asking price of Practice 1 is $1 million, which is below the capitalized earning market value of approximately $1.5 million, while the asking price of Practice 2 is $400,000, a price that is above its capitalized earning market value of $313,603.

Investment Yield Approach

The investment yield approach demonstrates the ability of the practice to potentially pay a dividend to the buyer. The investment yield can be determined by calculating the return on investment (ROI), which is the annual return divided by the initial investment (ie, the agreed-upon purchase price of the practice) (Table I-4). You can compare the ROI for the

Table I-4 Investment yield approach to valuation of hypothetical practices

	Practice 1 (Annual return = $380,000)		Practice 2 (Annual return = $80,000)	
	Purchase price ($)	ROI (%)	Purchase price ($)	ROI (%)
Highest price range	1,489,612	26	400,000	20
High mid price range	1,000,000	38	360,000	22
Low mid price range	800,000	48	313,603	26
Low price range	500,000	76	200,000	40

purchase of these practices and decide which—if any—price meets your investment objective based on your risk tolerance.

Summary

Based on the three practice valuation methods, the practice value range for Practice 1 is $500,000 to approximately $1.5 million and $200,000 to $400,000 for Practice 2. This is the range, also know as the *bracket*, from which to negotiate price.

The final purchase price depends on how motivated the buyer is to buy and the seller is to complete a transaction. If the seller must sell because of the onset of an unexpected health problem (ie, a fire sale), then he or she may be willing to sell at the lower price. If the buyer is willing to wait and look for another practice opportunity, he or she may walk away from the purchase opportunity rather than pay a higher price. So, the expert advice on the intrinsic practice value and optimum price is, "It all depends!"

Reference

1. Hill RK. Transitions: Navigating Sales, Associateships & Partnerships in Your Dental Practice. Chicago: American Dental Association, 2006:32–47.

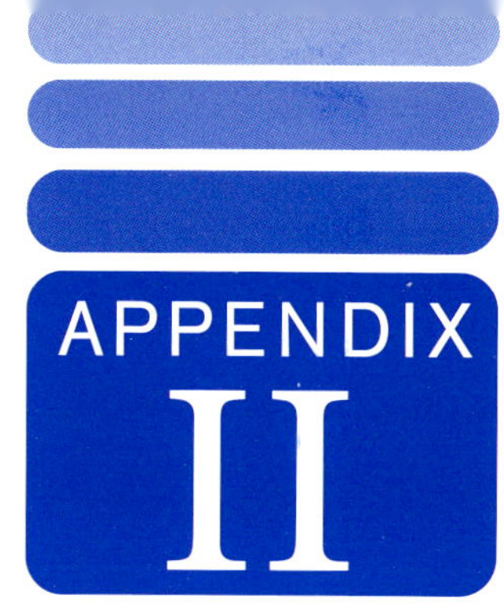

Sample Business Plan

Michael Okuji, DDS, MPH, MBA

The following business plan is based on the Business Plan 2 design presented in chapter 10.

Cover Sheet

Proposal for a Startup Dental Practice
1234 Market Street, Suite 1
San Francisco, California 94123

Michael M. Okuji, DDS
Room 23-086 CHS
10833 Le Conte Avenue CHS
Box 951668
Los Angeles, California 90095-1668

310-825-8574 (24 hours a day)
mokuji@dentistry.ucla.edu

September 1, 2014

Executive Summary

Michael Okuji, DDS, seeks a $300,000 dental practice loan to establish a general dental practice located at 1234 Market Street, Suite 1, San Francisco, CA 94123. The 1,200-square-foot, three-operatory office is located in a health professional building within the financial district, which is central to 200 large business firms within an 8-block radius. More than 50,000 commuters arrive in the area daily via the Bay Area Rapid Transit (BART) and the San Francisco Municipal Transportation System (MUNI), both of which have terminals directly in front of the building.

The new practice will focus on cosmetic dentistry and appearance-related procedures, and it will emphasize customer service and convenient office hours. It's expected to show a positive cash flow within the first 18 months with sufficient income to service the loan. Dr Okuji is a 2010 dental school graduate with an Advanced Education in General Dentistry (AEGD) residency certificate and 2 years of experience in a Valley Village, California, general dental practice.

Table of Contents

Mission Statement

Our mission is to provide competent, confident, and caring dental care in a timely manner. We believe in the three As of a successful business: affable, affordable, and accessible. Customer service is the hallmark of our office.

Vision Statement

Our dental practice will deliver high-end cosmetic and appearance-related dental care to 1,000 downtown San Francisco workers within 3 years.

The Practice

Michael Okuji, DDS, is a nonincorporated sole proprietor who plans to open a new dental practice at 1234 Market Street, Suite 1, San Francisco, CA 94123. The 1,200-square-foot suite, which had been occupied by a general dentist for 20 years, is plumbed for three dental operatories with a reception area, front office, laboratory, and storage space. It is situated in a 20-story, 50-year-old health professional building in the heart of San Francisco's financial district. The tenants are exclusively dentists, physicians, and allied health professionals. The 5-year gross lease is $2.15 per useable square foot for the first year with an option to extend for two additional 5-year periods. The owner plans to allot $15,000 for buildout and improvements.

Dr Okuji's primary focus is cosmetic restorative services, including veneers, invisible braces, white fillings, and teeth whitening, all of which are high-demand services in the financial district. Dr Okuji's dental school training was heavily weighted toward appearance-enhancing procedures. These skills were honed during his 1 year of AEGD training. In addition, his 2-year, full-time associateship in the Valley Village General Practice expanded his proficiency in endodontic, oral surgery, and periodontal procedures.

The Dental Market in San Francisco

More than 50,000 people commute to jobs at this locale every weekday. The BART and the local MUNI service the area and have terminals directly in front of the building. Retail, telecommunication, information technology, financial, legal, accounting, and small businesses abound within an 8-block radius, and NewCo Dental PPO, a large managed care company, enrolls back-office employees in more than 75 firms within the radius.

The financial district's commuter workforce prefers to access dental services near the workplace. This is a health-conscious group with high disposable income who seek upscale dental care as evidenced by a high demand for single-appointment teeth whitening, implants, all-porcelain restorations, and single-appointment computer-aided design/computer-assisted manufacture (CAD/CAM) crowns. Appearance-related dental service is not insurance driven and is paid in cash. The financial district doesn't attract patients with Medicare, Medicaid, or those covered by health maintenance organizations.

The Competition for General Dental Services

Thirty-five general dentists practice within an eight-block radius of 1234 Market Street. Their ages range from 28 to 63 years, with a median age of 49 years. After visiting each office and talking with the receptionists, I found that these dentists only practice 4 days or less each week and don't schedule patients before 9:00 am, after 5:00 pm, or during the lunch hour. These practices are closed 5 weeks per year for personal time off, and most have not introduced digital radiography, intraoral cameras, silent electric handpieces, flat-screen monitors, or other features that enhance the dental experience.

There are two orthodontists, three periodontists, two endodontists, and one oral surgeon in this neighborhood, all of whom practice at 1234 Market Street.

Marketing for a New Urban Dental Practice

Interviews of dental staff revealed that the local workforce is transient in nature with high turnover. A new worker relies on advertising and marketing efforts to find a new dental office with the features he or she wants, so the traditional personal referral from a friend or coworker is not as strong as direct marketing.

New patients prefer flexible office hours, convenient appointment times, short waits for the initial appointment, no waiting period in the reception area, and efficient treatment to lessen the number of visits required. This office will be open 5 days a week with early morning, lunch hour, and late afternoon appointment times to address these preferences. Front office staff members are trained with regular refreshers on how to effectively schedule appointments to allow for efficient treatments with no waiting in the reception area or the treatment rooms. Nitrous oxide and audio headsets will be standard for patients with longer treatment appointments. An office website is being constructed to facilitate marketing efforts. It will be updated monthly and provide access to dental health information, new procedures, general office information, and an "Ask the Doctor" feature to allow patients to ask questions.

External marketing will include wall and bench signage on the BART and MUNI terminals, which will be posted for at least 12 months. Dr Okuji will be listed on NewCo PPO's website, and his listing will include his extended office hours. All promotion will emphasize the patient experience, including convenient office hours, nitrous oxide availability, audio enhancements, and the state-of-the-art facility.

Customer service will focus on immediate telephone response, preappointment insurance verification, on-time performance, efficient treatment, and follow-up care, including postoperative telephone calls. Internally, cutting-edge digital radiograph imaging, intraoral and extraoral digital imaging, interactive patient education screens, and three-dimensional image design will be employed to engage the sophisticated patient. At the conclusion of every new consultation appointment, the patient will be given a printout of his or her radiography with notation, intraoral photographs, and a treatment plan. Pretreatment and digitally modified posttreatment photographs will also be given to those who seek appearance-related services.

The Management Team

Irene Kamafuji will be the office manager. She has 20 years of dental office management experience, including 10 years at a dental school. She will establish the financial policy, accounts receivable, accounts payable, communication network, website, and chart system, and she will ensure that the practice is compliant with the Health Insurance Portability and Accountability Act.

The dental assistant, Susan Gerski, holds a registered dental assistant license and has 30 years of dental office experience, including patient management issues. She will be responsible for clinical protocol, including Occupational Safety and Health Administration compliance, inventory, sterilization, imaging, and CAD/CAM technology, as well as patient care.

Cara Batson, RDH, will provide dental hygiene services on a limited basis for the first 6 months of the practice, then she will extend her services to 24 hours per week.

Legal service is provided by Gary Herman, Esquire, Valley Village, California. Accounting service is provided by Lee & Rappeport, LLP, Santa Monica, California. Both specialize in dental practice issues and already represent dentists within the building.

ABC Dental Supply Company will be the principal dealer to supply major equipment, supplies, and design services, and the company will install and maintain the equipment. ABC extends a discounted, just-in-time dental supply program that provides competitive prices and allows the office to maintain adequate supplies without a large inventory. ABC's office design studio has designed more than 50 offices of similar size and supplies blueprints for the contractor.

Contractor's Service Company (CSC) is the general contractor for the office buildout, and the company has remodeled 10 suites at 1234 Market Street; therefore, CSC is familiar with the building's systems. CSC obtains all permits and complies with local building regulations and the Americans with Disabilities Act requirements. CSC is uniformly on budget and on time.

Cash Need for the First 24 Months

A $300,000, 120-month loan will provide:

- $150,000 in dental equipment and supplies
- $85,000 for office buildout
- $30,000 in fixtures and furniture
- $35,000 in working capital

The location at 1234 Market Street will allow $15,000 for buildout that will be paid directly to CSC. The office will open for business within 9 months from the day of loan funding, allotting:

- 7 months for design and buildout
- 45 days for equipment installation, systems integration, and testing
- 15 days for employee training

Marketing and advertising will begin 15 days prior to opening.

Practice revenue is expected to grow from $200,000 for the first year to $300,000 for the second year. Earnings before interest, taxes, depreciation, and amortization are expected to rise from $28,000 in the first 12 months to $118,600 in the second 12 months of operation.

Pro Forma Financial Statements

Append the following statements (see chapter 10):

- Combined business and personal pro forma 24-month cash flow statement
- Business pro forma 24-month cash flow statement
- Personal pro forma 24-month cash flow statement

Appendix

Attach as many of the following documents as you have available:

- Equipment, instruments, and supplies estimate
- Furniture estimate
- Contractor's estimate
- Office lease, including leasehold improvements (buildout) allowance provided by landlord
- Blueprint of office space
- Resume
- State Dental License
- DEA License
- Professional liability insurance cover sheet
- Life insurance cover sheet
- Disability insurance cover sheet
- Business premises insurance coverage
- FICO score

- List of personal debt, including student loan, automobile loan, and credit card balances
- Federal Tax Return 1040 for the past 2 years
- W-2 wage statements
- Area map of local businesses
- Area map of competing dentists (generalists and specialists)
- Website homepage layout

Index

Note: Page numbers followed by "f" and "t" indicate figures and tables, respectively. Those followed by "b" denote boxes.

A

B

M

N

O

P

S

T

U

V

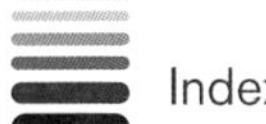

W